SIZE
MATTERS

SIZE
MATTERS

The Hard Facts About Male Sexuality
That Every Woman Should Know

Harry Fisch, M.D.,
and Kara Baskin

 THREE RIVERS PRESS • NEW YORK

Published in the United States by Three Rivers Press,
an imprint of the Crown Publishing Group, a division of
Random House, Inc., New York.
www.crownpublishing.com

Three Rivers Press and the Tugboat design are registered
trademarks of Random House, Inc.

Library of Congress Cataloging-in-Publication Data

Fisch, Harry.
Size Matters: The hard facts about male sexuality that every
woman should know / Harry Fisch and Kara Baskin.—1st ed.
Includes index.
1. Men—Sexual behavior.   2. Men—Health and hygiene.
3. Men—Psychology.   I. Baskin, Kara.   II. Title.
HQ28.F57 2008
613.9'52—dc22   2008002804

ISBN 978-0-307-40659-0

Printed in the United States of America

Design by Phil Mazzone
Illustrations by Nancy Heim

10 9 8 7 6 5 4 3 2

First Edition

CONTENTS

INTRODUCTION

KARA BASKIN:
I am a woman. Chances are, if you're reading this, you are too. And I, like you, have spent countless hours—commiserating with friends, chortling at how-to-date books, whining to therapists, roommates, coworkers—picking apart the seemingly capricious, confusing male mind. It can be a thankless task. Men mean mystery. For my friends and me, anyway, there are always behaviors that simply beg to be decoded: the way he speaks to a waitress at a restaurant; his voice mail greeting; the way he signs his e-mails; his Wii technique. Anything's up for analysis, and everything foreshadows something potentially wonderful . . . or something sinister.

Meanwhile, the male *anatomy*—something that can actually be scientifically explained—remains overlooked.

We're discriminating creatures. We wouldn't buy stocks without doing the proper research; or rent an apartment without scouting out the neighborhood; or begin exercising without mapping out a precise plan to demolish that excess ab fat. Shouldn't we do the same when it comes to our sexual lives? Be honest: When you're entering into a serious relationship with someone, you want to know everything about him. You Google him. You know where he works and maybe even how much he makes. You know the names of his last four girlfriends; you know all about his last bad breakup (the chick was psycho—you've determined this from stealthy Facebook stalking); and you know all about his childhood puppy, his embarrassing college roommate, and his meddlesome mom. You can talk late into the night about your favorite movies and books; you cook dinner together; you've met his friends; and you keep toothbrushes in each other's apartment.

But, ladies, do you understand his penis?

Outwardly, the male body seems so simple, of course. Guys don't have to worry about annoying things like periods. Their sexual organs dangle outside their bodies, arousal is easy to identify, and what you see seems to be what you get. But once you've dated enough, the plot starts to thicken. We all have our war stories: There's the dreamy guy with the semen that tastes like turnips; the sweet Emo guy whose penis curves terrifyingly to the right when erect; and that burly football player who couldn't get an erection at all. Untrimmed pubic hair; hairy balls; lopsided testicles. Each guy is a little weird in his own special way. And if he isn't weird? Well, that's weird too.

What does it all mean? In this book, we've tried to answer some of your most common and pressing questions about the male anatomy. These are things you'd probably never ask the man in your life. Most guys aren't burning with desire to talk about their ejaculation problems or masturbation habits, after all. And your friends might not be much help, either. Good information, like a good man, is hard to find.

This book is a fun, prescriptive, easy-to-understand troubleshooting guide for women who've spent oodles of time analyzing what's going on inside the male mind. What we really need is a book that tells us, smartly and humorously, what's going on inside a guy's *pants*. As such, you might ask why I, a woman with a husband and without a medical degree, am qualified to cowrite this probing chronicle of the male form. Good question. The same thing that could qualify any of you—because when it comes to unsatisfying sexual experiences, confusion, dating disasters, and nagging questions, I'm right there with you. Though I'm now happily hitched, I'm fairly well-acquainted with the male form (sorry, Mom; very sorry, Brian).

And let me be the first to tell you: Just because you've walked down the aisle, the Good Sex Fairy doesn't automatically sprinkle orgasm dust on your new Pottery Barn sheets. If anything, the stakes become higher. After a spate of bad sex, you can't just lose his phone number. If you're considering having kids, fertility questions come into play. And then there's the whole familiarity conundrum: After a man begins clipping his toenails and naming his farts in front of you, the mystique of romance really begins to fade.

Married or not, my girlfriends and I often blame ourselves when sex turns sour. We think, if the sex is bad, it must have something to do with a deep, meaningful, soul-shattering revelation about our relationship. He can't stay erect? Maybe I don't talk enough. Wait, maybe I talk too much! His libido is low? He's clearly offended by the fact that I make more than him—unenlightened jerk. Falls asleep after sex? I'm smothering him! It must have been those tampons I left in the bathroom. . . . Accuse me of offensive gender stereotyping, but each one of these statements has come directly from the mouth of a twentysomething female. Women often overanalyze. Men, well, don't.

And so I say: Ladies, rejoice. You are not at fault. Stop beating yourself up over bad sex! As you'll learn in these pages, thanks to the medical insight of Dr. Harry Fisch, there's actually a scientific explanation for most bedroom blunders. And these explanations have nothing to do with misplaced tampons. It's just that, more often than not, there's a real physical explanation for the things we attribute to psychological incompatibility.

This isn't to say that you shouldn't date guys with whom you're intellectually matched. But if your relationship is otherwise healthy save some sexual snafus . . . don't despair. Just keep reading. This book is intended to assure you that, no, sometimes the problem really is him—and sometimes the problem is easily solvable. Like you, I've dated men with whom I've clicked; like you, I've also languished in dead-end courtships too long, thinking that maybe, if only I behaved differently, was quiet when I was loud, loving when I was overbearing, I could change things. The only thing you need to change is your anatomical knowledge, my friends. Armed with the information this book provides, you'll have an educated idea of when to run, when to stay, and most of all, why things happen the way they do. And from better understanding will come better sex.

A word about my humble coauthor, the man who provides the answers in our fun-to-read Q & A format. Dr. Harry Fisch is a renowned New York urologist who's been seeing a parade of men in his office every day for 20 years. He sees men who struggle with fertility and erectile dysfunction, but he also sees guys who just want to know why their penis is behaving a certain way, or why their testicles hurt, or whether or not they're satisfying their partners. When Harry and I met, questions flew. Wouldn't it be nice, Harry and I thought, if there were a handy, fun-to-read, informative book about the male anatomy? We're not out to make light of sex, or to exploit guys, or to tell you how to please your "man" in seven seconds with the most mind-blowing orgasm of his life, glossy girlie magazine–style. There's plenty of that stuff out there. We believe women are smarter and deserve better.

Consider this book your own personal goodie-drawer road map to the male physique. Think of it as the sex-ed class you didn't get in seventh grade. You may never know why he's not that into you, but with our book, you'll finally understand him better when he's *in* you.

HARRY FISCH, M.D.:

How does a professor at Columbia University come to write a book titled *Size Matters*? Well, in addition to being a professor, I'm a urologist and a fertility doctor who treats men having problems conceiving a baby. I've become an expert in examining men and diagnosing problems with fertility and/or sexual performance—problems that are becoming more common these days as the average age of parents keeps rising. I have learned over the years that there are certain common "flags" of sexual problems. And one of those flags is the origin of the title of this book.

You see, one of the first things I examine in any new male patient is the size of his testicles. It turns out that the larger the testicles, the greater the likelihood that fertility, testosterone levels, and sexual function will be normal. On the other hand, the smaller the testicles, the greater the chance for infertility and sexual problems. This is definitely a situation in which size matters.

Here's the thing, though. As director of Columbia University's Male Reproductive Center, I frequently give lectures to medical residents about the diagnosis and treatment of male infertility. Usually, half of the audience is women. Very smart women. They've excelled through four years of college and four years of medical school, and are in their final stage of training. And yet, time and time again, I've found that neither they nor their male colleagues know about such seemingly simple things as the fact that, when it comes to fertility, the size of a guy's testicles is all-important.

Here's another example of something I've come to take for granted but that few people outside my profession seem to know: The size of a guy's belly is related to his testosterone level and, therefore, likely sexual performance. Men with large bellies (potbellies) tend to have low testosterone levels, for reasons I'll explain later. That's right, the fatter a guy is, particularly around the waist, the greater his chances for low fertility and erectile dysfunction.

These kinds of experiences were the germ of the idea for this book. Then I started asking women what they thought about the title. They all immediately thought I was talking about the size of the man's penis. One woman immediately raised her voice and said, "You're damn right, size matters!" Before I could tell her that I meant the size of the testicles or belly, other women jumped in with their own very vocal opinions. That's when I realized that "size" really does matter and that there was more to talk about here than just fertility.

At cocktail parties, I began talking about the book. Boom! I was suddenly the center of female attention. Women started pelting me with all sorts of questions regarding male sexual function. Then I started writing down the questions. I discovered that women talk about men and their sexual problems a lot. One woman said to me, "What did you think we talk about?" I had no idea. But I quickly realized that most women had very little understanding of male sexual health. That's a big problem, because if the man has a problem, the woman has a problem. Not only will both of them not be sexually satisfied, but the woman often feels responsible somehow. It's hardly ever the case, actually, but that seems to be a common emotional response. (Men aid and abet this, of course, with their prodigious capacities for denial and with their tendency to avoid talking about sex in general.)

Let me give you an example. Premature ejaculation is when a man ejaculates before a woman is satisfied. Many, many women have told me this happens all the time with them. Many said that they thought this was just the way sex is for guys. Well, not true. When I explained how long a man should last, they were astonished. And when I explained how they can help prolong the man's erection and prolong the time to ejaculation so that they could have an orgasm, they were thrilled. These are the kinds of explanations that can make a real difference in the quality of your sex life. This book is loaded with many more.

The more I talked to women about this book idea, the

more questions I was asked. How often are couples having sex? Does age affect sexual ability and by how much? Can you get a sexually transmitted infection if a guy wears a condom? Then came some questions that I did not expect. Why does semen taste the way it does? Why is it sweet or salty at different times? Why and how often do men masturbate? What are they thinking about? How does Viagra work? (And do you have samples you can give my husband?) One woman asked how often couples their age had sex. I told her that in her age group, the average was about twice a week. Her face dropped. "We only have sex about twice a month," she said. This told me that size and frequency matter. I informed this woman that what really matters is whether she and her husband were satisfied with how often they had sex. If not, there were plenty of things they might do about it—including checking to see if there were physiological problems going on with her husband that could be corrected.

The point, again, is that information can be empowering. It's ironic to me that we give "sex education" to kids in middle and high school, then let the adults fend for themselves. It's clear to me that despite early education (such as it is) and despite our sex-saturated society, most people really don't know enough about this most basic and potentially wonderful part of life.

So now you know how this book came about. It's not a book for guys. It's for you: an intelligent, curious woman who wants to know more about the male sexual machinery. Maybe you've had a few sex partners in your lifetime and you've seen enough variety to make you wonder why things are so different. Maybe you're worried about STDs and trying to be more careful when handling male body parts. Or maybe you're trying to get pregnant (or trying not to get pregnant!) and you want to know if there are any signs that the problem might lie with your partner (there are). Or maybe you're just curious about some quirk of male anatomy—why your guy's penis curves when it's erect, what sex and orgasm feel like for a guy, whether it's normal for one testicle to hang lower than the other. That kind of thing. Whatever your motives, I can guarantee you're going to learn something here.

Although I've written my answers to Kara's questions in a deliberately casual-sounding way, there is a great deal of medical and scientific rigor behind the answers. If no data exists to guide an answer, I'll tell you—and clearly say I'm giving you my opinion as opposed to facts. Most of the time, however, my answers are backed up by high-quality research. I provide a fairly extensive set of notes so you can dig deeper into a particular issue if you want. But a second purpose of the notes is to assure you that even when things sound bizarre, like my discussion of the flavors of semen, I'm not making this stuff up. Believe it or not, somebody, somewhere, has studied these things.

So that's it. The book is in question/answer format. If you have a specific question, you can use the index and go right to the topic that's tickling your curiosity. Have fun with this . . . and do me a favor—Leave it lying around where your partner is likely to find it. Maybe he'll read it and become one of those rare men who actually know how their body works—and how it can work better to pleasure you!

THE PENIS

The Measure of a Man

LADIES, TELL ME SOMETHING. How many times have you dated a guy with the highest of hopes, only to be unpleasantly surprised? Fess up. We all have some squirm-worthy skeletons in our closet: the Harvard M.B.A. with the pristine Cabbage Patch doll collection; the luscious guy from the gym who shaves every inch of his pubic hair and wants to be called Lucille in bed; the tormented musician who doesn't have a checking account because he gets paid in cash . . . for delivering pizza on his bike. The world is crawling with such creatures. While we can't single-handedly yank every deadbeat Lothario from the dating pool, we can spare you some surprises below the belt.

Let's assume you've avoided any doll- or bicycle-related pitfalls and have actually found a terrific guy. The time is right and the mood is set: fine wine, candlelight, rose petals

11

scattered on 600-thread-count sheets—and out bounces a penis that looks like a sausage link. Or, equally troubling, a throbbing purple mega-erection that could do more damage than an overzealous Pap smear.

When it comes to penis size, shape, color, and behavior, there's a lot of wiggle room. Some of these questions have come up during my own experiences, some are based on Dr. Fisch's real-life medical encounters, and still others have come to us from perplexed women who leapt at the opportunity to pose sticky questions in an anonymous forum. What's normal? What's not? When should you run screaming to the nearest nunnery? We're here to help.

Okay, Harry, let's start with the basics—penis size. This book, after all, is called Size Matters. *Why is there so much variation? Some are short and girthy. Some are long and pencil-thin. Pornography would have us believe that all men are hung like fire hoses. What's the average length of an erect male penis?*

☞ Ladies, readjust your expectations. Gentlemen, breathe a sigh of relief.

Average length is not as long as most people think. Scientific studies of the size of erect penises—and there are a surprising number of them—consistently show that the average erect penis is a little more than 5 inches long.[1, 2] Measurements (whether for science or curiosity) should be done on the top side of the penis from the tip down to the pubic bone at the base of the penis. The pubic bone is a nice, firm "stop" point on the top, while the underside of the penis has no natural "end." It is continuous with the upper part of the testicles. So no cheating, guys.

But I've come to believe that penis size varies on a man-by-man basis—remember that Seinfeld *episode? I think George Costanza gave voice to the insecurities of all men when he shouted, "I was in the pool!" It's sometimes kind of freaky to see a tiny, shriveled penis—makes you wonder how big it is erect. What's the normal size of an . . . unexcited penis?*

THOSE MACHO GAY GUYS . . .

Nobody really has an explanation for this, but several studies have found that homosexual men have, on average, penises that are about a third of an inch longer than those of heterosexual men.

Source: Hamilton, T. *Skin Flutes and Velvet Gloves,* St. Martin's Press, New York, 2002, pages 82–83.

☞ Any guy will tell you that the size of his penis varies a lot over time. That's because the penis is basically a sponge. (Actually, it's composed of three cylindrical sponges.) You can squeeze a sponge pretty small. As you saw on *Seinfeld,* cold water does that to a penis. And actually, to the testicles, too. They literally shrink away from the cold and try to get closer to the body so a guy doesn't lose heat (or freeze his balls off—literally). But the same guy whose penis looks like an umbilical stump after a swim in the ocean may look like John Holmes when he's just out of the shower. Then he'll be warm, his penis will be soft but filled with a decent amount of blood, and he'll look quite "hung."

So don't judge a penis by its cover. Data from the penis-measurers (can you imagine having that job?) show that the average flaccid penis is between 3 and 3½ inches long. Interestingly, the data also show that shorter flaccid penises tend to enlarge proportionately more during erection than do larger flaccid penises.[3] So you really can't judge a penis until you've seen (or felt) it erect.

SECRET MEASUREMENTS

Want to learn how long your partner's penis is without feeling like Bob Vila with a measuring tape? Unfold a dollar bill or any denomination of cash. Every bill is 6 inches long. How does your partner measure up to George Washington? Relationship tip: Always round to the higher number.

By the way, the width of this page is a little over 5 inches. How does he compare to it?!

Hopefully, when women are feeling penises, they are erect—or about to be. That said, all men are not created equal! How much variation is there in the size of erect penises?

☞ Okay . . . so the average is a little more than 5 inches. But as you ladies know, men vary. Wildly. On the small side of things, a guy is considered normal if his erect penis is at least 3 inches long.[4] On the long end of things, studies say anywhere from 7 to 8 inches is on the large side in study populations.[5, 6] Longer penises certainly exist, of course. In his book *Penis Size and Enlarge-*

ment: *Facts, Fallacies, and Proven Methods*, Garry Griffin provides the following estimates:[7]

➡ Only 15% of men have a penis longer than 7 inches when erect.

➡ Only 3% of men are bigger than 8 inches when erect.

➡ A 9-inch penis is found in 2 out of 1,000 men.

➡ Only one man in 10,000 has a 10-inch erection.

➡ Only about 5,000 penises in the world are more than 12 inches when erect.

When does a guy's penis start to grow into its adult form? Is the penis a guy has at 16 the same one he'll have at 30?

☞ The penis starts to grow at the same time that pubic hair begins to sprout, the testicles begin to drop, and the rest of the body begins to respond to the flood of testosterone released during puberty. As you probably know, on average, guys hit puberty a year or two after girls. But puberty happens at very different times for different people. The range for girls is between ages 9 and 14, while for guys it can be anywhere from age 10 to 17. The peak of the curve is somewhere near 13 for guys. Although I just said the guys "hit" puberty, it's actually a very gradual process until that day in a boy's life when he suddenly finds himself with a full-blown erection. Depending on his level of education, this can elicit responses ranging from "Wow . . . cool . . . finally!" to "What the hell is going on here?!?" Once a penis begins functioning in an adult way, it can become quite a fascinating toy and most guys will spend a fair amount of time playing with it, seeing how it works, and just enjoying the pleasures involved. The ability to have an erection doesn't necessarily mean a guy can start ejaculating. And if a guy's not been told how to do it, it may take some time to figure it out, by trial and error.

And chances are, once their penis does stop growing, many guys will probably start wondering why they weren't born like Ron Jeremy, right?

☞ It's true: Most guys are clueless and many are convinced their penises are smaller than normal. A study in 2005 illustrated this perfectly.[8] The researchers evaluated 92 guys who had come to their hospital clinic complaining of a "small-sized penis." Here's what the researchers found: Out of the 92 men, no one was abnormally short. They were all just overestimating average size. After getting some facts and figures, most of them were relieved.

SWEET REVENGE

Snicker, snicker: Why is it that guys care so much about the size of their penises? We don't go around wishing that our vaginas were bigger. Ask yourself this: If a guy told you your breasts were too big or too flat, chances are you'd be a little hurt, but mainly you'd be pissed off and think he was a jerk. But would it cut you to the very core? Probably not. But with men, penis size and ego seem to be one and the same, and there's nothing worse than telling a guy his penis is too small to satisfy. In fact, why not tell that jerk who said your breasts were too small that your ex had a penis twice the size of his? There's no better way to hurt a man. I'm not recommending this tactic, of course . . . I'm not the doctor here!

A lot of men may claim that they've never tried to measure their own penis, but I'm not so sure you should believe them all. There are no good data here, but I've had enough conversations with guys to know that it's pretty common, especially in the early years of adolescence. Just remember: If your partner is uncomfortable or sensitive about the size of his penis, be very reassuring. And it might help him to know some of the statistics I've provided here.

Why is it that guys care so much about the size of their penises? Women don't do this. I really can't recall the last time I strolled through my gym locker room, sheepishly comparing my clitoris to those of the women in my yoga class. Sure, we compare hips, thighs, butts . . . and just about everything else with our lady friends. But when it comes to our sexual organs, it seems like anything goes. Not with guys, though. How come?

☞ I'm speculating here. But think about it—males have been powerfully molded by millions of years of natural selection. Competition for females has been fierce—literally, life or death. So guys are incredibly aware of physical attributes—of both males and females. Any guy who stands out in any way that other guys think might be attractive to females is gonna be viewed as a threat. And it makes sense to guys that women might think bigger is better when it comes to penises. Like antlers or something.

The funny thing is, the fact that the average is 5 inches is proof that women don't care that much. Again . . . look at it from Darwin's point of view. If women really liked only big penises, then the guys with the big penises would be getting more women. Over a million years, this would have the effect of gradually increasing the average length of the male penis. So if big penises were really so cool to women, by now Nature would have seen to it that most guys would be hauling around penises they had to coil up like fire hoses.

What about guys with incredibly teeny penises—in other words, our ex-boyfriends? Do some guys really have minuscule penises, or is this just urban legend or wishful 20/20 hindsight?

☞ Yes, tiny penises do exist. The medical term is "microphallus," which pretty much sums it up. Men with penises that are shorter than 1½ inches long when flaccid and shorter than 3 inches when erect have a valid reason to worry. A penis this small may simply make intercourse difficult or impossible. The guy will constantly be "popping out" of a vagina. Incidentally, this isn't just a problem for romance; if a guy can't have sex with a woman, he can't father children either (without assistance). So it's a real problem . . . but it's also a rare problem. Much less common than most men think.

How about freakishly large guys? As much as women like to play down the attributes of their exes, at the same time, we're always trying to convince our current partner that his penis is the biggest we've ever seen—even if it isn't. That said, sometimes you come eye-to-eye with a python . . . and it's not always a nice surprise. Medically, can a man be too big?

☞ The quick answer is yes, a guy can be too big. And that's probably not a bad thing to let drop to your average-sized boyfriend or husband—they'll feel great!

The real answer is that "too big" is an entirely relative thing. Certainly, if a guy's penis is longer than a woman's vagina, then the tip of his penis is going to hit the woman's cervix—which can be painful. This isn't actually a very common problem, because vaginas are generally very elastic and, as we've seen, penises longer than 8 inches are rare. The real problem, more often, is that guys try to penetrate their partner before she is physiologically ready. I'm not just talking about lubrication, either, though that's awfully important. When a woman is fully aroused sexually, her vagina literally expands both in length and width. A guy with a larger-than-normal penis who tries to enter his partner too soon is going to hurt her. And there's simply nothing that kills an erotic moment quicker than pain.

Go back to the expanding vagina for a minute. I know this isn't a PC question, but will a woman who's dating, say, an Irish guy have to expand her vagina less than a woman who's dating a black guy?

☞ Not significantly. Alfred Kinsey and his colleagues, in their classic 1948 work *Sexual Behavior in the Human Male*, found that the average length of flaccid white penises was 4 inches; for black penises it was $4\frac{1}{2}$ inches.[9] But when erect, there was no real difference between the two races. Other studies since then have produced similar findings.

What about body type? Are larger or taller guys naturally more well-endowed?

☞ Nope. All of the scientific studies about penis size I've mentioned found no correlation between a guy's height or build and the size of his member. In Masters and John-son's classic studies, for example, the largest penis of the 312 men studied was about 5½ inches long when flaccid and it was hung on a guy who was 5 feet 7 inches tall and weighed 152 pounds.[10] The smallest penis, measuring just 2½ inches flaccid, was on a guy who was 5 feet 11 inches tall and weighed 178 pounds.

Fair enough, but what about the famous foot myth? Is it true that big feet equal big penis? And what about hands? You'd be surprised at how many women sneakily gaze at a guy's feet or pay careful attention when holding hands. One friend of mine swears you can tell how big a guy is by analyzing the length and width of his fingers, and his dexterity by the way he holds a fork. You see, Harry, this is why dinner dates are so popular.

☞ None of that is true, unfortunately. Sorry—I know that would make it easier for you to know for sure what you're going to get. Despite some serious attempts, no connection has ever been found between the size of feet, noses, thumbs, earlobes, or index fingers and the size of the penis.[11] Oh . . . and buttocks. No connection there either. This last one was only recently proven. In Nigeria, especially among the Igbo tribe, there is a firmly-held belief that a man's penile size can be predicted from his physique and the size of his buttocks, with people of small physique and flat buttocks likely to have long penile lengths. In 2006, some doctors at Nnamdi Azikiwe University in Nigeria decided to test the belief.[12] After measuring the butts and penises of 115 men, the doctors concluded that the belief was completely unfounded. No correlation between general physique and penile length was found. And rather than small butts signaling a big penis, there was a very slight correlation in the other direction, with the bigger-butted guys having, on average, slightly larger penises.

So is penis size more like baldness, a gene that comes from one side of the family?

☞ Let's back up a sec. First of all, it's a myth that guys inherit from their mother whatever tendencies toward baldness they may have. Baldness is controlled by a host of different genes, and the contributions of both parents are involved. The same applies to the penis. So, yes, the size of a guy's penis (like the amount of hair he has, or lack thereof) is determined by the genes he inherits from both his parents. Fortunately for all of us, there's no comb-over equivalent when it comes to penis size. Donald Trump has nothing to hide when he drops his pants—though I don't think we'd want to be around to see it.

Size is one thing—we don't want to sleep with guys who are too huge or too tiny, but it sounds like that's rare. But shape—that is quite another beast entirely. Occasionally, women encounter penises that curve in odd ways, and that makes sex an acrobatic endeavor. Some curve just a little bit, which isn't a huge deal. But some of us have seen penises that should be measured with a protractor. Is this some sort of condition, or is it just a normal penis variation?

☞ Many penises curve slightly, particularly when erect, and that's normal. But the super-curvy ones are a result of something called Peyronie's disease. We're not always sure exactly why this happens, but about 1 out of 100 men will develop small, hard lumps called plaques on their penis.[13] These plaques don't expand the same way that the rest of the penis does. When the penis is limp, you don't notice. But when the penis "inflates" the plaques cause the penis to curve in one direction or another. A plaque on the top of the shaft (most common) causes the penis to bend upward; a plaque on the underside causes it to bend downward. The plaque itself is benign, or noncancerous.

Symptoms may develop slowly or appear overnight. If the case is mild, it doesn't interfere with sex. But if the bend is severe—and I'm talking about nearly a right angle here—intercourse can be either painful or impossible. A variety of treatments can reduce or correct the problems.

What about more creative and deliberate ways to enhance the penis? I know that some guys like to spice up their penile repertoire with things like cock rings or penis pumps. Do these things really work?

☞ Depends on what you mean by "work." Vacuum devices and pumps are actually valid tools that some guys use for erectile problems. They put their penises in the tube, the air is sucked out (either by manual pumping or with a little battery-powered pump), their penis enlarges to its erect size, and then they slip a rubber ring onto the base of the penis to trap the blood inside. Cock rings do the same thing, except they come in a bewildering array of colors, shapes, and materials. They all serve the same purpose: As long as blood is trapped in the penis, the penis stays erect.

But there are some important things to think about here. One is that a tight ring of any kind around the base of the penis is going to compress the urethra—the tube that carries semen. The rubber rings used with prescription-grade vacuum devices typically have a little notch on the bottom specifically designed to avoid crushing the urethra. Sex-toy-grade cock rings usually lack this feature, which can be a problem. Rings without a urethral notch—or any ring that fits too snugly—can block the exit of semen. The semen may be forced backward in the urethra, up into the bladder. This "retrograde ejaculation" can be painful, though in most cases it isn't dangerous. The semen is expelled with urine the next time the guy goes to the bathroom.

But, women, think about this. Have you ever taken a rubber band and tied it around your finger? Notice how the part that's constricted gets slightly bloated and purplish from the blood that filled up there? When you trap blood in the penis with a ring, it cools off. Also, since

ASK A GUY

Do all vaginas feel the same?

A 25-year-old male replies:

No, they don't! They're all warm inside, but they can be wetter or dryer or looser or tighter. The wetter the better usually, but a loose, wet vagina can feel like having sex with an underwater cave—it's next to impossible to come. A tight, dry vagina chafes too much, and that's no fun for her either.

the blood is trapped only in the penis itself and not in the spongy "roots" of the penis, the penis is floppy. And a cold, floppy penis . . . well, you get the picture.

Cock rings vary. Some encircle just the base of the penis, and some are designed just to encircle the head. Some encircle the penis and base of the testicles, or just the testicles. Some incorporate vibrators of one sort or another that are designed to stimulate the man or his partner or both. Regardless of the design, it is prudent to select a ring with some kind of quick-release feature, because getting even a rubber ring off of an engorged penis can be difficult and/or painful. A warning: Falling asleep with a cock ring on can also be dangerous. Cock ring users should keep in mind that any pain, discomfort, or feeling of coldness in the genitals is a signal to take the cock ring off. Cock rings must not be used by those who have cardiovascular problems, by diabetics, or by those who take any blood-thinning medications.

What about those guys who insist that wearing a condom is like an anti-cock ring—a surefire erection-killer? Is this true or just a lame excuse? Why can't a condom be more like another sex toy?

☞ Any condom will definitely diminish the sensitivity of the penis. It feels a little like being slightly numb. This can actually be a good thing for guys who tend to ejaculate very quickly. Wearing a condom can slow him down, and this is one relatively easy thing to try as a remedy.

But as far as I know, no condom is going to make a healthy guy lose his erection. And, these days, some condoms are very thin and don't diminish sensation significantly. Unfortunately, thinner also means easier to break . . . and that could be bad news indeed!

Especially if the guy in question is too big for his condom. Which brings me to this question: Can guys get penis extensions? Women can get bigger boobs, bigger lips, tighter vaginas. Do guys have the same options? Are all those e-mails for "penile enhancement" for real?

☞ If the e-mail is for some herbal supplement, forget it. Nothing he takes by mouth is going to make a bit of difference to the size of a guy's penis. (Of course, some things, like Viagra, will affect his erections, but even drugs can't do anything about its actual size.) Sometimes vacuum devices are sold as "penis enlargers." As I just mentioned, these devices will certainly enlarge a guy's penis while it's in the vacuum chamber. But it's a bit difficult to have sex with the thing on your penis! And no permanent enlargement is produced by these devices. In fact, they can be dangerous. Create too much suction and you're gonna start breaking blood vessels in the penis, which will leave the guy with a really ugly-looking penis and possibly scar it on top of that, which could really impair his erections.

The only valid forms of enlargement are surgical— and you're only a candidate for these if you truly have a tiny penis, the "microphallus" I described earlier. One type of surgery releases ligaments at the base of the penis, which lets it hang down farther and appear longer. Other types of surgery use injections of natural or artificial materials to "bulk up" the girth of the penis. All of these carry risks common to any surgery—except we're dealing with an exquisitely sensitive organ here, so the pain of recovery is, well . . . really painful.

How about natural enhancement through exercise? Will a rigorous gym routine change the shape or size of a penis in the same way that working out can change the shape and size of a woman's breasts?

☞ If that were true, you'd see a lot more guys in the gym. But, no—the penis doesn't have any skeletal muscle that can "bulk up" with exercise. Nor can "exercising" the pubic muscles around the penis have any effect.

But if a guy exercises enough to lose belly fat, the result could greatly improve the appearance of his penis simply by uncovering it. There's actually a name for when a guy's belly or pubic fat obscures his penis—it's called "buried penis syndrome." It's pretty common these days, because we're in the midst of an obesity epidemic. But if an overweight guy loses the fat, his penis is going to "emerge" and look a good deal larger than it did before.

Let's assume for our purposes that our readers have unearthed their partner's penis and are ready to begin the subtle art of pleasuring it. Is it true that the head of the penis is the most sensitive part?

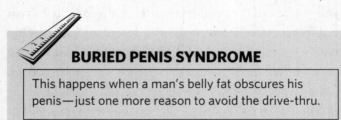

BURIED PENIS SYNDROME

This happens when a man's belly fat obscures his penis—just one more reason to avoid the drive-thru.

☞ It's difficult to generalize about this—and certainly difficult to study objectively. If masturbation techniques are any indication of which parts of the penis are most sensitive, then the only thing one can say is that every part can produce pleasurable feelings. Masters and Johnson report a diversity of masturbation techniques in men, with some men using only a very light touch on the bottom of the penile shaft, some confining their stimulation to the head of the penis, and others using a very forceful pumping of the entire shaft with only minimal stimulation of the penile head.[14]

One of the most sensitive parts of the penis is the foreskin, which is commonly removed in infancy in this country via circumcision. The foreskin has a richer variety and greater concentration of nerve receptors than any other area of the penis. Consequently, circumcision strips a guy of a part of his body endowed with tremendous pleasure-generating nerve cells. Of course, he won't miss anything because he's got nothing to compare things with and, by and large, what's left is still more than capable of providing pleasure. But his untrimmed brethren are experiencing a quality and degree of sexual pleasure that he can only imagine.

Is the penis head's mushroom-cap appearance designed with pleasure in mind?

☞ That's a great question—and I wish I had an answer for you. The fact is, I've never come across anything about this—aside from numerous observations that the penises of many mammals share this mushroom-cap design. Since the purpose of the penis is to deliver sperm, the subtle flare of the head of the penis (technically called the corona glandis) may act to limit the sperm from exiting the vagina too rapidly. The more important feature of this part of the penis is the opening (called the urethral meatus). The opening should be at the very tippy-top of the penis. It isn't completely unusual for the opening to be set some distance back from the tip—a condition called hypospadias. The more severe the hypospadias, the more likely that sperm will not be efficiently placed at the cervix and the greater the chance that the man will have difficulty getting a woman pregnant.

Does foreskin add length to a penis? What about sensation for a woman?

☞ On some men, the uncircumcised penis in its flaccid state has a tiny "turtleneck" of skin at the tip that would make the penis appear very slightly longer. But more often, the foreskin doesn't completely cover the penis tip and so doesn't add any length. Once the penis is erect, the foreskin pulls back and the head is exposed, so it looks and feels similar to a circumcised penis. The extra skin of an uncircumcised penis can "slip" along the shaft of the penis more easily than the skin of a circumcised penis, which can be noticeable by a woman.

Snipped or not, is it normal for a guy's penis to stick straight out when erect, or should it be "saluting" at a higher angle?

☞ The "angle of the dangle" depends mostly on the age of the guy. Generally, the younger the guy, the higher his penis will "stand." With age, the erect penis droops, though it is still perfectly functional in all respects. Here's a handy (pardon the pun) way to visualize the "ages of the penis":

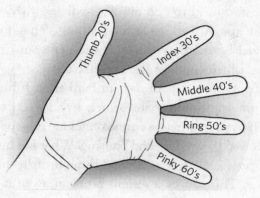

Decades of a Man's Erection Angle

Since the penis is so sensitive and it gets hard like a bone, does that mean it can break? My husband is always cringing during Three's Company *reruns when there's a reference to any sort of injury to the nether regions.*

☞ Surprisingly, yes, the penis can break. Sort of. Unlike some animals (walruses and some whales, for example), human males do not have a penis bone. This is a good thing. Most of the time, a penis needs to be out of the way and safe. (Soft and squishy is perfect.) Having a literal "boner" constantly would definitely make this more difficult.

But, obviously, sometimes the penis needs to be very rigid indeed—more bonelike, in other words. This is accomplished by some very sophisticated plumbing and some amazingly expansive, spongelike tissue that runs the length of the penis. Basically, if you open up the spigots of blood feeding the penis, the sponges are quickly pumped full of blood by the pressure generated by the heart. But sponges alone do not a hard-on make. You also need to contain the sponges with something quite tough, inflexible, and strong. That function is served by the outer layer of the penis, just under the skin, which contains ligamentlike tissue.

So if an erect penis is bent hard enough by an errant thrust, the unfortunate owner, in addition to yelping with pain, may hear a curious cracking or popping noise, followed by swelling and bruising. What has happened is properly called a "fracture," though of ligaments, not bone. This can be a serious problem, even if the penis appears to heal. The scar tissue that can form after a penile fracture can cause Peyronie's disease, which causes the penis to have a bend to it that can be annoying or even debilitating.

By the way, the sexual position that involves the most serious risk of penile fracture? Woman on top. This is probably because in this position it's very easy for the woman to rise up a tad too high during thrusting, thus letting the penis slip out. If it slips all the way out, it's cause for a momentary readjustment. But if the penis is almost, but not quite, all the way out and the woman thrusts back down quickly . . . well, that's when the snap, crackle, and pop is more likely to happen.

Let's forget about length and sensitivity for a moment and talk about girth. Many women will tell you that it isn't the length of the penis that matters, it's the width. When we say that size matters, this is what we mean!

☞ A recent study—one of the first on the matter—seems to back up your hunch.[15] A random sample of 556 women who had at least some experience with intercourse were interviewed about their preferences when it comes to penises. Whereas 102 women said the length of a man's penis was "very important" to them, 120 women said the girth was "very important." Roughly the same number of women (140 and 142, respectively) felt that neither length nor girth was important.

Does a veiny penis indicate anything other than healthy blood flow?

☞ No. It may not be the prettiest of organs, but there's nothing abnormal about it.

What about weather conditions and climate? Do guys living in Alaska tend to have smaller penises than guys in Hawaii?

☞ Geography is not at all correlated with penis size— though temperature certainly is. Other things being equal, a guy standing in his boxers outside in Alaska in January is going to have a much shorter-looking penis than will a guy in boxers on a Hawaiian beach. Just remember that there's very little correlation between the size of a cold-shriveled penis and its length and girth when erect.

Can a penis get permanently small? What would cause a penis to shrink—not temporarily, but for good?

☞ A side effect of a variety of illnesses (uncontrolled diabetes, for example), medications (estrogens or testosterone-reducing drugs), and some types of prostate surgery is something called "penile atrophy." This doesn't mean the penis literally shrinks, it just means that the penis loses its ability to enlarge. A penis that is always in its normally compressed, small state may appear to be permanently small, but that's just because it's no longer getting large on a regular basis.

A girlfriend of mine felt a lump on her husband's penis. Should she be freaked out that he's cheating on her and got a sexually transmitted infection (STI)? Or has cancer?

☞ Maybe freaking out isn't necessary, but concern is certainly warranted. It's unlikely that the lump is cancer, though he should see his doctor ASAP. More likely, the lump is either a lymphatic thrombosis (meaning a clog in a lymph vessel), a hematoma (blood-filled swelling resulting from injury), or a plaque of the type that causes Peyronie's disease. Of course, it could also be a genital wart—which is a form of STI and which might be more of a reason to freak out (unless she is a carrier of the virus that causes the warts, of course).

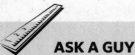

ASK A GUY

Do you ever sneak a peak at another man's penis in the gym shower or at a urinal?

I try not to. In fact, there's an entire bathroom urinal etiquette: Stand close to the urinal, head forward or straight down. No turning or talking. The gym is different. It's hard to avoid seeing sometimes, but I'd rather not.

HARD FACTS ABOUT THE PENIS

Size of the average American penis: 5.4 inches

Average diameter of erect penis: 1.5 inches

Average increase in penis length upon erection: 63%

Average increase in penis circumference upon erection: 32%

Size of an average hot dog: about 6 inches

Animal with the largest penis: The penis of a male blue whale is almost 10 feet long and a foot in diameter.

Smallest human penis ever recorded: five-eighths of an inch

Largest human penis ever recorded: 13.5 inches

Longest known erection: Men with a disorder of erection called priapism may have an erection that lasts several hours. Far from being a badge of manhood, however, this is a medical emergency. Blood in an erect penis cannot circulate and be refreshed with oxygen. If the erection is not medically "doused," a man with priapism may suffer permanent damage to his member, which, in severe cases, will require amputation.

Farthest measured ejaculation: 11.7 inches

Animal that produces the most ejaculate: blue whale—4 gallons per ejaculation.

Sources: Hamilton, T., *Skin Flutes and Velvet Gloves,* St. Martin's Press, New York, 2002, pages 61 and 66. Simmons, M. N., Jones, S. T., "Male Genital Morphology and Function: An Evolutionary Perspective," *J. Urology,* 2007; 177(5): 1625–1631. Arnott, S., *Sex: A User's Guide,* Dell Publishing, 2003.

I'M JUST A LOVE MACHINE

How Sex Drive Works

ALL RIGHT, LADIES. NOW it's time to discuss the hugely important topic of libido. Pop culture dictates that men are, by and large, horny creatures who think about sex all the time; dream about bulbous breasts and lesbionic trysts (often involving Uma Thurman); and spend the better part of their teenage years nursing a constant hard-on. Of course, this stereotype is unfair—we've all had boyfriends with less sex drive than we have, and my husband really doesn't understand the hype about Uma—or so he says.

Still, by and large, men do seem to be able to get turned on much more easily than women. But one male friend of mine, an otherwise intelligent and enlightened fellow, recently commented that he could gear himself up to have sex with any woman, so long as it was dark enough that he could pretend he was with a Spanish model with long, dark hair and a sultry accent. (If that's all it takes, I'm cutting up my Victoria's Secret credit card, getting a Clapper, and never wearing makeup again!) Another guy confessed to me that he thought about sex every few seconds, and even had a trick for snapping himself out of badly timed naughty reveries: picturing Margaret Thatcher splayed out naked in a tub of butter. Are men really sex-crazed Neanderthals? Is your boyfriend's "but I'm at my sexual peak!" excuse for sleeping with a Vegas stripper really valid? Is your cubicle-mate currently picturing a cholesterol-drenched prime minister? Harry, please enlighten us.

First things first, Harry: horniness. If a guy's ready to have sex all the time, does that mean he's bubbling over with testosterone like a luscious fondue?

☞ Probably. Testosterone is the hormonal fuel of the sex drive—aka libido—in both men and women. Broadly speaking, the more testosterone, the higher the sex drive. (Note, though, that women have only a small fraction of the total amount of testosterone in their bodies that men have.) In fact, horniness is probably the one "marker" of testosterone level that has some accuracy. Others, such as physique, profession, athleticism, and baldness, are all notoriously poor predictors of testosterone levels. In other words, a light-framed mathematician who hates sports can easily have more testosterone—and a more ferocious sex drive—than a burly firefighter whose idea of fun is bagging a buck and celebrating with his buddies by watching the game at the local bar.

One study of testosterone levels in men of different professions—actors, ministers, football players, physicians, firefighters, professors, and salesmen—found one statistically significant difference in average testo-terone levels. Ministers' average testosterone levels were on the low end, and both actors' and football players' averages were on the high end.[16] But every group displayed wide individual variations—some football players had lower testosterone levels than some ministers, and some professors had higher testosterone levels than many firefighters.

What about the opposite problem? Is there any way to tell if a man is suffering from low testosterone?

☞ You bet! Just look at a guy's waist size. In general, the larger the waist, the lower the testosterone. That's because testosterone is normally broken down in the body's fat cells. If you've got a lot of fat, in other words, your body breaks down testosterone extra quickly,

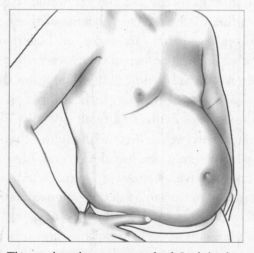

This man has a low testosterone level. Look familiar?

a deficiency. And it turns out that abdominal [38] "belly fat," has a greater capacity to convert ...terone to estrogen than fat stored elsewhere, such n the limbs or buttocks.

mm. That's good to know. I would have thought that a bulky guy naturally had more testosterone—I'm flashing back to the Don Juans on my high school football team. Is there such a thing as a natural, normal amount of testosterone?

☞ This is an interesting question. Not really. Unlike, say, blood pressure or body temperature, both of which have relatively specific values for "normal," it turns out that there's a huge range of "normal" when it comes to testosterone. Any level between 300 and 1,100 nanograms per deciliter of blood is considered normal.[17] Although guys on the low end will probably have a less intense sex drive than guys on the high end, they'll both be perfectly "functional" in that regard and you wouldn't be able to predict their T level just by looking at them. It's only when guys have either very low or very high testosterone levels that physical or mental changes are noticeable.

Men with levels below 300 (a condition called hypogonadism) tend to have little interest in sex and are usually nonconfrontational, socially inhibited, and physically weak. Men with higher-than-normal testosterone tend to be just the reverse: obsessed with sex, competitive, aggressive, extroverted, physical, and tending toward more action-oriented activities or careers. But within the normal range, testosterone levels play only a background role and other aspects of personality dominate.

What about bald guys? Is it true that, by some feat of biological justice, hair-free men have higher testosterone levels?

☞ Ever since the Samson myth, there seems to have been a connection between hairiness and testosterone-fueled machismo. So it's a little surprising that science has found a clear association between a lack of hair and higher levels of testosterone.[18] It turns out that hair follicles (on the head, at least) respond to the levels of two male hormones, testosterone and dihydrotestosterone (DHT). But the hormones inhibit the follicles rather than stimulate them. Several studies have found a correlation between higher levels of these hormones, particularly DHT, and a tendency toward male-pattern baldness—that's the "classic" type in which the hairline recedes from the forehead and from the top of the head down.

The connection between testosterone and hair loss can also be seen in the side effects of some medications. Some drugs used to treat prostate problems, for example, block DHT. Men on these drugs often find that their baldness stops getting worse (though they don't grow any new hair). On the other hand, men given testosterone supplements often find their hair loss accelerating.

While dating a balding man certainly isn't ideal for some women, worse yet is a woman with a healthy sex drive dating a man who has a low testosterone level. If a guy is low on testosterone, can he regain his sexual youth by taking testosterone supplements?

☞ First of all, testosterone isn't taken as a "supplement." Testosterone is destroyed in the stomach. That's why it has to be either injected or slowly infused through the skin with a gel or a patch. Second, testosterone is like gasoline—it's easy to blow yourself up with it (figuratively speaking). If a normal guy uses a patch or gel, he may very well feel a stronger sex drive or feel "younger." But he may also make himself infertile. High doses of testosterone are actually a fairly good male contraceptive! In addition, testosterone can spur the growth of existing prostate cancer cells. Only if a guy has truly below-normal testosterone should testosterone replacement therapy be considered—and then only under the care of a doctor.

In terms of a testosterone timeline, for lack of a better term, are guys at their sexual peak when they're teenagers?

☞ From a purely physiological standpoint, yes. Whatever way you measure physical sexual response, the young guys are gonna win, whether it's speed in attaining an erection, ability to maintain the erection, libido, or ability to regain a new erection following ejaculation. When it comes to testosterone levels, the "peak" is actually later—around 20.[19] When men are in their thirties, testosterone levels begin an inexorable slide of about 1 percent a year—which can add up after a while.

So if all you're looking for is a robust penis, by all means rob the cradle. As with wine, though, you simply cannot get the best, most delicious, complex, lingering, subtle flavors in a young man. Older men have more experience in pleasing women, for one thing. Add to that the fact that young guys are much more apt to ejaculate very quickly, and you get plenty of reasons to reject the

"younger is better" line of reasoning. A lot of wom[en]
prefer their wine with a little age.

I know many guys tend to be at their most "robust" first thing in the morning, regardless of age. Why is that? Does this mean they wake up wanting to have sex?

☞ Many hormone levels in humans (and other animals) vary on a daily basis. Testosterone levels vary as well, with peak levels tending to occur in the early morning, dropping significantly by midafternoon. This is an average, of course—some men's "cycles" will be flatter than others. And younger guys may not notice anything because their T levels are high enough that they're basically horny all the time. But this daily "wave" of testosterone can become more apparent with time. Maybe you should learn to surf!

Guys often wake up with erections because they've been sleeping with erections. Technically, this is called nocturnal penile tumescence. On a typical night, a guy will have a series of erections having nothing to do with his dreams. (Though, of course, men have sexual dreams, and these dreams can certainly induce erections and/or ejaculations.) These erections are the body's way of keeping the penis healthy.

In its normal flaccid state, a penis doesn't get much blood flow. It can't; otherwise it would be erect—and that's just not a very comfortable or handy state to be in all day. To keep the penis flaccid, the arteries leading into it are shut down to a trickle. That means there's not a lot of oxygen getting to the tissues and not a good current of blood to remove metabolic waste products.

solution? Open up the valves at night and
tem with nice, fresh blood. Typically, the
us while this housecleaning is going on—
many ways our bodies take care of them-
.....out us having to worry about every little
detail.

One interesting note about this phenomenon is that
nocturnal erections are an excellent way to determine
if a guy actually has erectile dysfunction. If a guy comes
into my office and says he can't get an erection to
make love to his wife, well . . . the problem could be a
whole lot more complicated than his plumbing. One
way to determine if the problem lies in the meat or the
mind is to measure nocturnal erections. If the guy's got
perfectly normal erections at night but can't get it up
with his wife, he doesn't need a pill, he needs some
therapy.

*So there's a daily cycle to testosterone levels. Makes sense. What
about monthly? Do guys have a testosterone version of a woman's
period?*

☞ No. Nature appears to have designed the male reproductive capacity to be ready at all times with only relatively minimal fluctuations in testosterone and sperm
production. Since sperm are very cheap, from a physiological point of view, there's no reason to create them in
any type of cycle—whether weekly, monthly, or season-
ally. (It had been thought that testosterone varied in a
seasonal way, but more recent and rigorous research
finds no such seasonal variation.[20]) On the other hand,
it's a big deal, physiologically speaking, to prepare a

woman's uterus and her egg for possible fertilization, and hence the need for a relatively long fertility cycle in human females.

I know some women who just aren't huge fans of sex. It's not that common, but it doesn't seem that odd, either. Talking, cuddling, just hanging out watching a movie can be really exciting for a woman because of the closeness it provides. But men are "supposed" to be constantly sex-ready. Or are there guys out there who don't care about sex either?

☞ Like every other stereotype, the one labeling all guys as sex-obsessed is cartoonish and wrong. Like practically everything else in nature, sex drive falls on a continuum. Yes, some guys really don't care about sex. Generally speaking, these are guys with very low levels of testosterone. That's relatively uncommon in younger men, but it does happen for a wide range of physiological reasons. It's more common in older men, whose testosterone levels are naturally lower than they once were. Guys who were on the low end of the "normal" spectrum of T levels when they were young may well find themselves going for days at a time not thinking or really caring about sex when they're in their fifties, sixties, or older. That, too, is normal. It's Nature's way of taking their sperm cells—which are much more likely to be damaged or unhealthy—out of the gene pool. Of course, there are plenty of older men who most definitely have a sex drive, and there's absolutely no reason they can't continue to enjoy sex as long as they want (barring obvious medical conditions such as serious heart disease).

What about guys who can get it up but can't seem to fertilize their wives? Everything seems fine, erections are normal, the guy gets aroused looking at his wife (and not just a stained copy of Jugs magazine)—yet the sperm don't seem to be swimming in the right direction.

☞ There's a big difference between wanting sex (libido) and being able to father children (fertility). Testosterone is mostly involved with libido. If a man wants sex and is having sex regularly, testosterone is not the problem. If a guy isn't fertile, the problem is much more likely to involve his sperm. And, by the way, a lot of women think that if they're not getting pregnant, there's got to be a problem in their plumbing. That's dead wrong.[21]

In about 40 percent of infertile couples, the problem lies with the man. In the same percentage of couples, it's the woman who has the problem, and in the remaining 20 percent either both partners contribute or the cause is unknown. About 10 percent of men trying to conceive a child—roughly 2,500,000 men in the United States alone—are either infertile or subfertile. Many of these men don't know they have a problem yet, mainly because they haven't been tested. So their problem remains undetected and medical attention shifts to the female.

My husband likes to tease that the average guy thinks about sex every seven seconds. Is this true? If not, how often do men fantasize about sex?

☞ Depends on age. One study revealed that most teenage boys think about sex at least several times an hour and as often as every few minutes. Studies of sexual fantasies routinely demonstrate that men fantasize about sex much more often than do women.[22] As I just noted, as men get older, their sex drives decline and fantasies about sex get replaced with daydreaming about open tee times and clearance sales at Home Depot.

Or else they're trying to regain their hard-on. Judging by the frequency of Cialis commercials, it would seem every man over 50 has erectile dysfunction. (And sits on his front porch, holding hands with his wife, staring vacantly out toward the horizon.)

☞ Erectile dysfunction is the persistent inability to get or maintain an erection. The largest study done to date estimates that between 20 million and 30 million men in the United States experience some degree of erectile dysfunction, the incidence increasing steadily with age.[23] About half of men in this study who were between 50 and 60 reported some erectile dysfunction. The percentage increases to 60 percent at age 70, and 70 percent at age 80 and above.

So, no, not every guy has this problem—though the drug companies might wish that were the case. The fact is that Cialis, Viagra, and Levitra are all being used very widely, and not just for the guys with a true plumbing problem. Of course, as long as the pills are used as prescribed, there is probably only a small risk of problems. But the risk isn't zero. These pills can sometimes trigger an erection that won't quit—a condition called priapism after the Greek fertility god Priapus, mentioned earlier. In priapism, the blood is literally trapped in the penis, and that's a very bad thing. I'll spare you the gory details, but let's just say that prolonged priapism leads to scar tissue within the penis that results in complete loss of erections.

Some guys with constant hard-ons aren't modern-day incarnations of Priapus, but claim to be sex addicts. My trusty Us Weekly *always seems to carry a tale of cheating based on sexual compulsion— Charlie Sheen, anyone? Could these guys actually have an addiction problem?*

☞ Sex addiction exists, but if these guys are sex addicts, so are a couple of billion other guys. Seriously—for better or worse, "cheating" is epidemic among men and women. Recent studies reveal that 45–55 percent of married women and 50–60 percent of married men engage in extramarital sex at one time or another during their relationship.[24] And that's just for married couples. People in nonmarried relationships are perhaps even more likely to have an affair, so the prevalence of cheating is probably even higher than these numbers.

Sexual addiction (or "sexual dependency") is a valid disorder, however. Like any addiction, sexual dependency is a compulsive behavior that completely dominates one's life. Sexual addicts make sex a higher priority than family, friends, or work. They are willing to sacrifice what they cherish most in order to preserve and continue their unhealthy behavior.

No single behavior pattern defines sexual addiction— and it has not yet been given a formal listing in the *Diagnostic and Statistical Manual (DSM)*, the bible of diagnosis used by psychiatrists.[25] But generally speaking, the behaviors that can be engaged in by a "sex addict" include: com-

pulsive masturbation, compulsive heterosexual an
mosexual relationships, compulsive viewing of porn
phy, prostitution, exhibitionism, voyeurism, inde
phone calls, child molesting, incest, and rape.

Oh, dear. I'm glad most guys have simpler desires. Not that their preferences aren't confusing: Why are some men "ass men" and some men "breast men"? Why aren't there any "elbow men" looking for love on Craigslist? Why isn't "Baby Got Back" called "Baby Got Arms"?

☞ Men are "ass men" because all our male primate cousins are "ass men." Primates (monkeys, apes, baboons, etc.) mate from the rear. Nature has therefore tuned men to be extremely perceptive about all things derriere. In many primates, the female genitalia become visibly reddened or swollen or otherwise changed when she's in heat. So it pays to pay attention to that part of the body and not, say, elbows.

The male attraction to breasts may have slightly more complicated roots. Certainly, it's plausible that men have an inborn interest in breasts because they are a sign that a woman is (a) old enough to bear children and (b) capable of nursing those children. But breasts are also very primal structures—for men and women—because most babies are, at least for a little while, sustained by them. To a baby, a breast is Mother—the source of comfort, warmth, food, and drink all rolled into one. I know of no studies looking for a connection between the length of time a man was breast-fed and his preferred erotic interests as an adult. But it's dimly possible there would be a connection there.

It's worth noting, however, that what men find erotic also has a strong cultural and learned component. In eras and cultures in which women were almost entirely clothed all the time, necks and ankles or shins became highly eroticized. Likewise, the body types and shapes considered beautiful have varied widely over the centuries and still vary today among cultures.

Okay, so is this why men get unexpected erections? They happen to catch a fleeting sight of cleavage and just can't control themselves?

☞ Random erections are a very common (and embarrassing) problem for teenage guys. Their penises and scrotums are so sensitive that the rubbing of underwear or the vibrations from a car or other vehicle can set off a raging erection—it's not necessarily a glimpse of an erogenous zone that does it. Even the most fleeting of fantasies can do the same thing. It's all just a hypersensitivity that Nature builds into the scheme of things to maximize the chances for successful mating. Of course, try to tell that to the kid who's having a devil of a time rearranging to best conceal his boner in a high school math class.

Concealment seems to be a theme when it comes to men's sexual tendencies. I was dusting the other day and came across a lesbian sex DVD in my husband's sweater drawer. I guess it's better than DVDs of bronzed men prancing around in thongs, but still. My husband denies that he's attracted to lesbians, but then he's always joking with his friends about sapphic Swedish bikini models and some famous scene from the movie Wild Things. *What is the appeal?*

☞ File this under "Questions Yet to Be Scientifically Investigated." In the absence of data, I'll offer my informed speculation. Men are frequently attracted sexually in a purely physical way—love's got nothing to do with it. Women can be attracted in the same way, but they do tend to be more picky about their sex partners. This, of course, has to do with some fundamental biological facts, such as how relatively precious a woman's eggs are compared with the zillions of sperm a man casts out on every orgasm. And the fact that a pregnant or nursing woman is very vulnerable and, thus, more motivated to look for males that might stick around to help out and provide some protection.

But this choosiness on the part of women says something. It communicates a sense of caring for the chosen sex partner. This may or may not actually be true—we no longer live in caves and women can now avoid pregnancy if they want. But, still, there's an unavoidable aura about women and sex that implies caring and an emotional connection.

So when two women are making love to each other, men may very well sense or infer that the women actually like each other in a way that a man may (or may not) like his sex partner. Perhaps this inference of emotion adds an additional layer of interest or resonance to the experience of a guy watching a female/female coupling. That, or guys may simply be curious. Novelty can be titillating, after all, and, at least when first exposed to lesbian sex, the sheer difference may be riveting. Another possibility is that no penises are involved in lesbian sex—no real ones, anyway. Some guys just don't like watching other penises do their thing.

How many times can a man at his sexual peak have intercourse in one day?

That depends on whether—or how often—he ejacu-
ates. Men who practice Taoist sexual techniques learn
to control their ejaculation in order to maintain an erection for as long as they or their partner desire. In fact,
ejaculation is not considered the "goal" of sex, from a
Taoist perspective, and ejaculating during every act of
intercourse is discouraged. If the question is how many
times can a man ejaculate in a single day . . . well, more
than three or four, but nobody's really studied this to my
knowledge. After ejaculation, the penis usually loses
some or all of its stiffness and is unresponsive to further
stimulation for a period of time, known as the latency
period. This can range from only a minute or so for
teenagers to several hours for older men. With repeated
ejaculations, the latency period lengthens until no
amount of stimulation will elicit a response. When a guy
hits this ultimate wall, however, is highly individual and
very difficult to study scientifically.

The advent of erection-enhancing drugs such as Viagra has enabled men to "turn back the clock" to some
extent, giving them a shorter latency period and allow-
ing for more prolonged intercourse.

*Fine. But let's talk numbers here, Harry. How many times a week do
men really want to have sex?*

☞ That depends on their testosterone levels. Men with
higher testosterone levels have a higher libido and desire
sex much more often than men with lower testosterone
levels. How often? It probably ranges from two or three
times a day to once every couple of days—but, again,
nobody's studied this carefully to my knowledge.

Are men hornier at particular times of day or days of the month?

☞ As I've mentioned, for healthy young men, testosterone levels are highest in the morning and lowest in the early evening. But desire to have sex is complicated by many factors, such as available partners and social and work-related stress. So while testosterone may be high in the morning, the desire to have sex increases when there's a partner around.

Do men still get uncontrolled erections beyond their high school years? I swear there's this one guy on the subway who always seems to have tented trousers....

☞ Absolutely. Erections can be triggered by physical rubbing or vibrations, daydreams, memories of prior sexual encounters, and sexually stimulating images, smells, or sounds. But the frequency of "uncontrolled" erections normally wanes with age as a guy's testosterone level slowly drops.

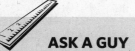

ASK A GUY

Do men often fantasize about sex with coworkers?

It's hard not to. To paraphrase Hannibal Lecter: "We covet what we see every day." Okay, maybe that's a little creepy. Even if we only think about sex a few times every hour, we're at work most of the day. It's hard *not* to fantasize about a hot coworker.

HARD FACTS ABOUT SEX DRIVE

Average number of times a man will ejaculate in his lifetime: 7,200

Average number of erections per day for a man: 11

Average number of erections that occur while a man is sleeping: 5

NUT CASES

Pearls of Wisdom About the Family Jewels

"GROW SOME STONES!" "MAN, you have cojones!" "Protect the family jewels at all costs!" "If my girlfriend blue-balls me one more time, I'm sleeping with her sister." Ah, the testicles—an integral part of everyday parlance, yet little understood. Guys are always scratching them, rearranging them, shifting them from one side to the other, protecting them from harm. Women, on the other hand, tend to overlook the balls. Many ladies I know are oblivious when it comes to the original man-purse: One close friend actually spent her teen years thinking that the balls were two large, separate sacs that grew from either side of the penis. But even if you didn't fail seventh-grade sex ed, chances are there's plenty you've yet to discover about the testicles. While the penis is important when it comes to sex, procreation, and all that good stuff, the testes are just as vital—if not more so—when it comes to sexual performance and function. We received countless questions about low-hanging balls, blue balls, lopsided balls, and overheated balls. So let's get down to nuts and bolts, shall we?

Let's begin with the (not so) obvious: Why do men have balls? What do they do besides hang there?

☞ We should start with what they don't do, which is store semen. Contrary to popular belief—even among guys— the testicles aren't where semen is kept and they don't participate directly in orgasm. The testicles are the male version of ovaries—in fact, they are "built" from the same basic embryological tissue that ovaries are. And, just like ovaries, the testicles make hormones and sex cells—in this case, testosterone (primarily) and sperm cells. But whereas women are born with all the eggs they'll ever have, guys start making sperm around age 13 and never stop (barring disease, of course). Making any individual sperm cell is actually an elaborate process that takes about two and a half months. Nonetheless, a healthy guy will pump out several hundred million sperm every day for his entire life.

Given the importance of testicles to the survival of the species, you might think it would have been wiser for Nature to tuck them well inside the body, just like ovaries. Unfortunately (especially for guys who play contact sports), the testicle factories need to be air-conditioned. Yep—the sperm-making machinery simply shuts down if it's raised up to normal body temperature.

They need to literally swing in the breeze to keep them cool. (Unless it's already cold out, in which case the scrotum contracts to hug the testicles close to the body.)

So why do men live in fear of anything thwacking them in the balls?

☞ The need for cool conditions during sperm production also means there can't be any armor around the testicles— so they're basically just sitting ducks for baseballs, elbows, and an infinite range of intentional or unintentional blows. And because the testicles are extremely well endowed with nerves, these injuries can inflict excruciating pain that can shoot up into a man's innards in a quite literally sickening way. Vomiting is common in guys who have suffered a hard blow to the testicles.

As we women have compared notes, we've found that there are all sorts of different kinds of balls—shorter scrotums, bigger nuts, lopsided sacs. Are there normal sizes for balls? Is it better to have bigger (or smaller) balls?

☞ This is probably the part of the male package where size definitely matters. And bigger is better. A normal testis is oval-shaped and at least 1.5 inches long and 1 inch across. It should be approximately the size of a walnut. (If you don't want to measure, there's another way—put four of your fingernails together like you're checking the nail polish. Four of most women's fingernails, measured together, are about 1.5 inches across—that's the size of a normal testicle.) When felt (gently!) through a loose scrotum, as you'll find when he gets out of a warm shower, the testicles will feel very smooth and will slip around a little inside the scrotum.

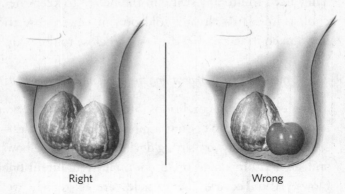

Right   Wrong

Soft or small testicles are a bad sign—in fact, this is one of the first things a doctor will check for when doing a fertility workup. If what you feel is more like a pair of Bing cherries or two large olives, then your man's on the small side. Likewise, any unusual hardness or lumpiness could be bad—possibly testicular cancer or some other testicular malady.

But the basic fact of life here is that bigger testicles mean more sperm and (probably) more testosterone. Which translates into a guy who's both horny and fertile.

I SWEAR BY MY BALLS . . .

In centuries past, it was common practice for men to hold their genitals when taking an oath. The Latin word *testes* in fact means both "testicles" and "witness." The words "testify," "testimonial," and "testament" all derive from *testes*.

At what age do a guy's testicles begin to "drop"? Does this happen during puberty or at birth?

☞ Until puberty, a boy's testicles are small and generally held fairly tightly in the scrotum. Bathed in the testosterone flood of puberty that they themselves make, the testicles enlarge, the scrotum develops, and the testicles "drop" into the adult (relaxed) form. And, as noted previously, the age at which this happens for guys is anywhere between 10 and 17, with 13 being about average.

Assuming a man's balls drop at the typical time, let's talk about fertility. I've heard rumors that soaking in hot tubs and Jacuzzis are bad for balls—especially if you're trying to get pregnant. Is this true?

☞ Yup. If you're trying to get pregnant, perhaps you should skip the balmy climes. Soaking in a hot tub for a half hour or so is going to temporarily shut down sperm production. Not a big deal if it's only done once in a blue moon, but if you're having a hard time getting pregnant, avoid romantic interludes in hot water.

And, by the way, fever has the same effect—which is why guys going to get a sperm count are told to wait for up to three months if they've had any kind of cold, flu, or infection that results in a high fever.

How about slightly asymmetrical balls—will that affect sperm count? If a guy isn't feng-shui perfect, could this cause problems?

☞ Nah, that's probably normal. In about 85 percent of men, the left testicle hangs a bit lower than the right because the thick spermatic cord supporting the left testicle is slightly longer in most men than the cord on the right—for reasons unknown.[26] But the difference in the way the testicles hang should be very slight. If it seems exaggerated, then the abnormal descent could be caused by a set of distended blood vessels on one side of the scrotum, called a varicocele (VAR-i-ko-seal). A varicocele, disgustingly, feels like a "bag of worms" inside the scrotum. They vary in severity. Many men have minor varicoceles and never even realize it. Others are large enough to cause problems with fertility, because the extra blood warms the testicles, which hurts sperm production.

Is it weird for those lopsided balls to change shape—during an erection, for example?

☞ This is an involuntary reflex. The testicles are raised and lowered via a muscular interior rope called the spermatic cord. As sexual tension builds, the cord tightens, reaching maximum contraction during ejaculation. Depending on the pace and nature of lovemaking, a guy's testicles may rise and descend several times as the sexual stimulation ebbs and flows.[27] Typically, a guy's testicles will rise and stay in that contracted state just before he ejaculates.

On the subject of big balls—can they be too big? One reader describes her husband's balls as "looking like a purse carried by Nicole Richie."

☞ You've actually just given a very good description of a relatively common testicular disorder called a hydrocele.

A hydrocele is a buildup of a watery fluid in the scrotum.
It can be caused by a number of things, including physical injury, infection, or congenital deformations of some
of the interior structures of the testicle. Hydroceles are
not usually painful and in most cases don't seem to interfere with fertility.[28] But because they are sometimes
caused by testicular cancer, any man with these symptoms should see his doctor pronto.

*Assuming cancer isn't an issue, though, is there a correlation be-
tween having big balls and, well, "having balls"?*

☞ Not much, mostly because "having balls" in the sense of
being a risk-taker probably has more to do with brain
chemicals (such as dopamine) than with testosterone.
Guys with unusually big testicles may also have high
testosterone levels and thus may be more prone to aggressive behavior, but that's not quite the same as "having balls."

*What about "blue balls"? Every guy I know insists that it happens—
and happens painfully—when they're aroused and then denied. But
in our earlier chats, you've laughed at this malady. Is it just a way for
guys to get sympathy and, hopefully, more sex?*

☞ Obviously, testicles don't become sky blue. But the term
does describe a real—if rare—phenomenon in some
men. In all my years as a physician, I have never seen a
patient complain about this phenomenon, mostly because it's a temporary problem and not a real medical
condition that requires treatment. Very little is written
about "blue balls" in the scientific literature, but we

have some idea of what's probably happening. Semen is produced by the seminal vesicles. The semen makes its way to the prostate to be ejaculated. If ejaculation does not occur, there is a buildup of semen that can cause pain near the scrotum or in the area of the prostate. This excessive semen buildup can also cause back pressure to the testicles. The remedy is obvious: The guy needs to have an orgasm, which triggers the release of the semen that created the problem in the first place. There's certainly no justification for a guy using "blue balls" as a lever to have sex, and no woman should feel the least bit concerned, since he'll just masturbate to relieve the feeling and probably enjoy himself in the process.

Okay, so the balls are sensitive and sometimes they hurt. Does that mean guys don't like to have their balls touched whatsoever?

☞ On the contrary. It's definitely erotic. Caressing or stroking a man's testicles is usually quite pleasurable, and guys may (or may not) do this themselves when masturbating. Given the sensitive nature of the testicles, there is a fairly thin line between pleasure and pain, however, so proceed with caution.

Why are balls covered with hair (in some men more than others— yikes)? What evolutionary purpose could that possibly serve?

☞ The prevailing theory about this relates to pheromones—those musky scents that both men and women produce during sexual arousal. In this theory, the tufts of hair that grow on and around the genitals, as well as under the arms, capture and disperse these erotic scents.

For some people, scents from these areas are very noticeable and pleasurable, and they consciously increase sexual arousal. Others either can't detect the odors or don't find them attractive. Whether they are consciously detected or not, however, pheromones can influence how we react and behave toward another person.

Hair on the genitals probably also serves a basic physical function related to friction. Hairs act like a dry lubricant—which is very handy in the tight quarters in which genitals (both male and female) typically find themselves. You can discover just how helpful hair is in this respect by shaving it off—the resulting friction can cause pretty painful chafing if you're not careful.

Some guys have an overabundance of pheromones—they stink down there. Musky is one thing. But nothing is worse than a gamey duck-hunting smell when the mood is set for romance. How can a man keep his testicles fresh and inoffensive?

☞ Daily washing and normal hygiene! Of course, some men perspire more than others, and that may mean more or less washing is needed to keep things smelling healthy. As we've seen, some men have a condition called varicoceles, which are excessive veins in the scrotum. These veins heat the testicles and cause increased scrotal perspiration—which means they'll require more frequent cleaning. (But that's the least of his problems—varicoceles can also cause the testicles to shrink and can result in infertility.) But if your partner smells bad all the time, he may have a basic grooming problem.

Would a guy rather a woman touch his penis or his testicles? Assuming, of course, that he smells nice down there.

☞ The testicles are definitely an erogenous zone with plenty of pleasure-producing nerve endings. But the penis, particularly the head of the penis, is even more richly endowed with these nerves. So it's possible that some men do derive more pleasure from stimulation of their testicles than their penis—but it's probably not a big percentage. The thing to remember here is that the scrotum and testicles are extremely sensitive to pressure. Just a slight squeezing can be uncomfortable or painful. Particularly sensitive are the structures that sit on top of each testicle, called the epididymis. (Some men have a condition called epididymitis, an inflammation that makes the epididymis so sensitive that even the slightest pressure causes discomfort. If that is the case, the guy should see a urologist pronto.) So the moral is, you gotta be more gentle with the testicles than the penis. Fondle, caress, but please don't squeeze.

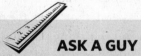

ASK A GUY

Why do some men prefer boxers and others briefs?

I can't speak for other guys out there, but I do know that because I wear a lot of flat-front pants and jeans, rather than pleated pants, I have to wear briefs or boxer briefs underneath. Otherwise, if I wear boxers, my crotch would look like a couple of oranges swinging around in a plastic grocery bag.

PUTTING TESTES TO THE TEST

We ladies are lucky—the importance of breast self-exams has been drilled into our heads and more and more women are making a point of checking themselves every month. If your partner doesn't do the same with his testicles, offer to help him out.

He should check his testicles monthly in the following manner:

- Do the self-examination lying in a warm bath or while having a long shower, as this relaxes the scrotum, making it easier to feel the testicles inside.

- Examine the scrotum, looking for any lumps, spots, or sores on the skin.

- Cradle the whole scrotum and testicles in the palm of your hand and feel the difference between the testicles. They should feel the same size and weight, though one typically hangs slightly lower than the other.

- Examine each testicle in turn, then compare them with each other. Use both hands and gently roll each testicle between thumb and forefinger.

- Check for any lumps or swellings. Both testicles should be smooth except where the duct that carries sperm to the penis, the epididymis, runs. This lies along the top and back of the testicle and normally feels slightly bumpy.

HARD FACTS ABOUT BALLS

Average size of male testicles: about 1.5–2 inches long and 1 inch wide

Average size of bull's testicles: roughly 14 inches in diameter

Percentage of men born with undescended testicles: 3–5 percent. As high as 30 percent in premature babies. In about 75 percent of such cases, the testicles will descend on their own within three months of birth.

Most extreme case of scrotal malformation: An African man suffering from the parasitic disease elephantiasis had a grossly enlarged scrotum 2 feet in diameter and weighing 154 pounds.

Source: Taran, I., Hartke, D. M., and J. S. Palmer, Congenital genitourinary anomalies and sexual function. *International Journal of Impotence Research*, 2007; 19:115–118.

SEX WITH SOMEONE YOU LOVE

Masturbation

IT SEEMS LIKE MASTURBATION is a way of life for guys, as natural and wholesome as football games and beer. I still remember learning about nocturnal emissions in my sixth-grade health education class. The girls and boys were separated when we learned about gooey lady stuff like periods. But when it came time to talk about boys and their graduation into manhood, we were thrown together and presented with this bit of information: Once a guy wet his sheets in the night, we were told, he could then begin to masturbate. Presto: He was a sexual being! The girls all looked embarrassed. I was still practicing kissing with my Laura Ashley pillow, for God's sake. The guys, however, all sat up a little bit straighter. Score!

A couple of weeks later, I was playing at a friend's

THAT FIRST ORGASM

Do you remember your first orgasm? What were you doing? Was it a surprise or were you *trying* to come? Not many scientists have asked these questions in a rigorous way, but Dr. Alfred Kinsey and his colleagues did. Here's what he found out:

Sources of first ejaculation for males:

68% masturbation

13% nocturnal emission

12% coitus

4% homosexual contact

3% other sources, including premarital petting

Sources of first orgasm for females:

40% masturbation

27% coitus

24% premarital petting

5% nocturnal dreams

3% homosexual contact

1% other sources

house. Her garage was actually a ramshackle barn, which her parents used for storage. It was there, stuffed behind some old gardening tools, that we came across stacks and stacks of dusty *Playboy* magazines addressed to her dad. Mouths open wide, we leafed through each one, page by

page, horrified and intrigued. Her dad had seen nal
women? He actually got magazines devoted to that very
subject? Our worlds were turned upside down.

That was 15 years ago, and all that's changed is the
technology. Just about every guy I know owns pornography,
looks at pictures of silicone-enhanced cyberseductresses,
and has a rotation of women whom they think about when
they do the dirty deed. While my women friends usually
need a glass or two of wine, a hot bath, and an extended
fantasy to get in the mood, it seems that all guys need are
an Internet connection and a free hand.

Some women I know think of masturbating as cheating,
especially because men don't often think of their wives or
girlfriends when they do it. I'm not being cynical: I've
heard this from countless guys, who claim to have a
"lineup" of women composed of ex-girlfriends, coworkers,
strangers from the gym, pillow-lipped former math teach-
ers, and, for those born in the 1970s, Princess Leia. They'd
never masturbate to their wives or girlfriends. "It's almost
kind of an insult to think of your wife that way," one
thoughtful husband told me. "I just fantasize about random
chicks for a few seconds. My wife is the one I actually have
sex with." Oh, so that explains it.

So let's attempt to confront the mystique of male masturbation. It's so easy! They do it so often! How do they
snap into the mood so quickly? Why can't we? And what
do they do with all that semen?

When do guys usually start masturbating?

☞ Before they're born. I'm serious! Although it's mostly a
reflexlike behavior, boys in utero have been "seen" via

ultrasound to manipulate their own fetal penises. This behavior continues after birth, and even infant boys can have baby erections (though, obviously, no ejaculation or orgasm). Boys "play with themselves" pretty much their entire lives, in other words. But if you restrict the meaning of "masturbation" to "self-stimulation to orgasm," then the answer is that guys start masturbating very near to the time that puberty has progressed enough to allow erections and orgasm. And that means anywhere between ages 10 and 17.

THE ORIGINAL MASTURBATOR?

In the Bible's Book of Genesis is the story of Onan, a man who practiced *coitus interruptus* as a way to prevent pregnancy. God was so pissed off that Onan "spilt his seed upon the ground" that He struck him dead.

Over the years, the fact that Onan wasn't actually masturbating was neglected or ignored and the term "Onanist" was used to describe anybody, male or female, who masturbated.

How do guys masturbate? Are there certain, um, techniques? Or is it more of a universal reflex?

☞ The most common male masturbation technique is simply to hold the penis with a loose fist and then move the hand up and down the shaft until orgasm and ejaculation take place. But Masters and Johnson noted pronounced variation in masturbatory techniques in their subjects.[29] Some men used only a very light touch on the underside of their penis, while others "use strong gripping and stroking techniques that for many individuals would be quite objectionable, if not painful."

Some men only stimulate the head, or glans, of the penis. If a guy is uncircumcised, his foreskin will slide back and forth over the glans. This gliding motion reduces friction. For guys without a foreskin, the contact between their hand and the glans is direct, and thus a lubricant is sometimes used to reduce friction.

Some guys like to masturbate in the shower, where they can use soap or shampoo as a lubricant. A less common technique is to lie facedown on a comfortable surface such a mattress or pillow and rub the penis against it until orgasm is achieved. This technique may or may not include the use of a vibrator or some kind of artificial vagina. Stimulation of the anus, with or without penetration with a finger or object, is another variant of normal masturbation.

One aspect of masturbation that is quite common regardless of the specific technique is that the rhythm of stroking increases as ejaculation nears, then decreases or even stops during ejaculation itself. Just after ejaculation, the glans of the penis can be exquisitely sensitive (as can the clitoris just after a woman's orgasm) and so men will often involuntarily protect the glans from further stimulation, whether after masturbation or intercourse. You'll be doing a guy a favor, in other words, to be extra cautious with any kind of bodily contact with the tip of his penis right after he comes.

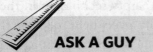

ASK A GUY

What do guys think about when they're pleasuring themselves?

A 27-year-old male replies:
   If I don't have porn in front of me, I'll think about a past hookup or ex-girlfriend. Or I'll fantasize about having sex with a coworker on her desk or with a friend's girlfriend in a bar. It's all fantasyland. No harm, no foul. Anything goes.

Okay, but . . . what about all that semen? Isn't male masturbation a pretty messy affair? What do guys do? Catch it with their free hand or something?

☞ Not unless there's no other alternative. How a guy deals with his ejaculated semen depends on his technique and preferences. If a guy masturbates in the shower, the problem is taken care of. If he's in bed, then he'll either just ejaculate on himself and wipe up afterward with a tissue or something, or, if he's a slob, he'll ejaculate on the sheets and let it dry there. If he's masturbating into something—a condom, a sock, or some kind of device— then he'll either clean up afterward or just toss the thing in the trash. Fortunately, semen is water-soluble, so it washes out relatively easily, even when dried on.

Harry, that would make a fantastic detergent commercial! "When my husband masturbates into his socks, just a quick spin in the wash and presto—good as new!" What about frequency? I've heard guys masturbate every day. This seems a little bit excessive, guys I've talked to don't seem to think it's that weird at all.

☞ I'm with the guys on this one. Daily masturbation? Not weird at all. How often a guy masturbates depends on three things at least: his age, his testosterone level, and how often he has nonmasturbatory sex. Other things being equal, young guys masturbate more often than older guys, high-T guys masturbate more than low-T guys, and guys who aren't having a lot of sex masturbate more than guys who are "getting it" on a regular basis.

What's typical? Some teenage boys may masturbate every day, and sometimes two or three times a day. A recent study of undergraduate men found an average frequency of masturbation of about three times a week. Another survey found that single guys who are in a relationship masturbate half as often (roughly once or twice per week). Of course, these are averages for healthy guys. Sickness, fatigue, and high stress can all cause a guy to stop masturbating at his usual frequency.

Even men who are in sexually satisfying relationships? I can understand a guy who's sexually frustrated masturbating all the time. But what about guys who are actually getting laid?

☞ Masturbation among couples in a sexual relationship is very common. A recent study found that nearly 85 percent of men and 45 percent of women who were living with a sexual partner reported masturbating in the past year.[30] Let's face it, people simply aren't always horny at the same time. Masturbation is the perfect solution. Of course, if you find yourself having more fun masturbat-. ing than having sex, maybe it's time to take a hard look at the relationship!

WILD MASTURBATION

A very wide range of male and female animals have been observed to masturbate. The list includes:

- Horses
- Bulls
- Goats
- Sheep
- Camels
- Elephants
- Kangaroos
- Porcupines
- Nearly all primates

  Indeed, female apes and monkeys have been observed fashioning dildos from sticks or bark, with which they stimulate themselves.

Source: Bagemihl, Bruce, *Biological Exuberance: Animal Homosexuality and Natural Diversity.* St. Martin's Press, 1999.

Let's talk about this "fun" concept for a second. Women love to go into sex shops and laugh at all the different jumbo-size vibrators—and sometimes we need them! Guys seem to have it a lot easier. Do they use accessories, too?

☞ The range of objects used to enhance or facilitate male masturbation is immense. Some of the more pedestrian:[31]

➡ Plastic bags filled with a lubricant like Vaseline
➡ Socks
➡ Bubble wrap
➡ Condoms
➡ Toilet paper rolls

You get the picture.

Then there are "toys" specifically designed for male masturbation. There are zillions of artificial vaginas sporting such fetching names as "Silicon Snatch," "Pocket Pussy," "Fleshlight," and "Pussy Palm Pal." There are also anal dildos, life-size inflatable dolls, cock rings, vibrators, and, of course, a wide range of lubricants.

"Fleshlight"—my favorite Parliament song! So let's say a guy has his Pussy Palm Pal in one hand and his penis in the other. How long does it take him to orgasm?

☞ The famed sex researcher Alfred Kinsey found in his studies that the average time to reach orgasm in men when they masturbated was between 3 and 4 minutes.[32]

This all seems so easy. It takes women much longer to masturbate— which is why we probably don't do it quite as often. Plus, you always hear old wives' tales about guys who masturbate too much—they'll grow hairy palms or go cross-eyed. Is it really possible for a guy to masturbate too much? (I secretly wish you'd say yes!)

☞ Medically speaking, it's extremely unlikely that a man will injure himself by masturbating too much. Even the most virile young penis will stop responding after a series of four or five ejaculations. After that, as they say, it'll be like trying to hammer a nail with a fish.

Of course, it's certainly possible to injure oneself by engaging in masturbation that involves sharp, hard, or suction-based objects or toys. As noted in a previous chapter, an erect penis can "fracture" if it is forcibly bent. Not only is this intensely painful, but it can also leave permanent scars that can induce curvatures of the penis in subsequent erections (the previously mentioned Peyronie's disease).

But there's a potential psychological hazard to masturbation as well. Men who use masturbation as their main form of pleasure grow accustomed to the arousal states associated with solo sex. This can take a variety of forms. For example, since a man can stimulate himself exactly as he wants, he may become accustomed to a relatively rapid transition from erection to ejaculation. Rapidity, however, is often an undesirable thing when making love to a partner. A penis (and brain) that has been extensively "trained" to ejaculate rapidly during masturbation may be harder to "slow down" during real sex.

What about the reverse? Can men have trouble ejaculating during sex if they masturbate a lot?

☞ Yep. On the other hand (so to speak), if a man becomes extremely familiar with a particular masturbatory technique, he can retard ejaculation during sex and/or promote erectile failure. The problem here is that the sensations and external stimulation of a partner may be very different from those accompanying masturbation. In a sense, the penis gets confused—it's no longer sure what's going on. And a confused penis is usually a limp penis, or a penis that can't ejaculate. (In medical lingo, this is called "retarded ejaculation.") Men who suffer from this find it hard to ejaculate with a woman, even though they have no problems ejaculating while masturbating.

There are ways to combat retarded ejaculation. If you suspect your husband or boyfriend might suffer from this, first you should talk to him about it. Ask him what excites him and what would help him achieve more excitement with you. Another method doctors use is to have the man change his usual masturbation technique. Most men know what gets them off, and they use the same technique again and again. If you have him vary his technique (use the left hand instead of the right, for example), he will not be so at ease with the routine and will learn to achieve arousal and climax on a variety of terms.

A friend of mine asked this question: "I've heard that some guys do something called 'prostate massage' while they masturbate. This sounds kind of disgusting. What is it?"

☞ The prostate gland is about the size of a walnut and sits below the bladder. It produces some of the fluid that

THE KINKY SIDE OF MASTURBATION

Although most guys use the standard masturbation technique of pumping their erect penis with their hand, there's a nearly infinite number of abhorrent ways in which some guys amuse/stimulate/pleasure themselves, which can lead to physical damage. Do *not* try this at home!

- Inserting a thin rod of wood, metal, or plastic into the small hole (urethral opening) at the tip of the penis.

- Using electrical stimulation devices to deliver pulses of electricity in varying patterns to the base of the penis or testicles.

- Piercing the penis shaft or head with metal studs of various shapes to produce mildly painful sensations during masturbation.

- Immersing the testicles and/or penis in warm or even hot oil, then using the oil to reduce friction during subsequent masturbation.

- Inducing a bee, or bees, to sting the penis, thus producing swelling and pain that, for some masochists, enhances the pleasure of masturbation.

makes up semen. During orgasm, it contracts rhythmically to help propel semen out of the penis.

Some men find that gently stroking or rubbing the prostate gland enhances their sense of orgasm. As any guy who has had a prostate examination by their doctor knows, the best way to feel the prostate is by inserting a finger into the anus. The prostate rests against the front wall of the rectum, so it can be felt as a smooth, firm lump there.

Prostate massage simply means inserting a small object—like a finger or toy—in the anus about 2 or 3 inches (some kind of lubrication should be used, since the anus does not produce any type of natural lubrication). Some people find prostate massage very stimulating; for others it's neutral, and for some people it is painful.

ASK A GUY

What is the greatest number of times you've masturbated in one day?

My friends and I were joking about that once. One buddy had done it 10 times. I think my penis would fall off after 7 or 8. In high school, you're so horny, some days you think to yourself, "All I really want to do all day is masturbate." But after a few times, your body starts to get over it.

HARD FACTS ABOUT MASTURBATION

Percentage of men who masturbate: between 90 and 95 percent

Age at which most men begin masturbating: At puberty, which can be anytime between age 10 and 15. Note that prepubescent boys, and even babies, can "play with themselves" and may even get an erection, though there is no ejaculation.

Most common places to masturbate: No data here, but you could plausibly conjecture the following: bed, bathroom, shower, and, these days, wherever the computer is.

Hand that most guys use to masturbate: Right for "righties," left for "lefties," though guys can and do switch hands to vary the sensation and/or give the "pumping" hand a rest.

Health benefits of masturbation: None known—the Taoists consider it unhealthy to masturbate frequently. There may be mental benefits, such as stress reduction and relaxation.

STICKY SUBJECTS

Coming to Terms with Semen

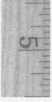

DO YOU LIKE THE taste of semen? Me neither. It's like the R-rated version of Forrest Gump's box of chocolates: You never quite know what you're going to get. It's sometimes salty, sometimes kind of sweet, and all sorts of viscous—kind of like a failed home-ec recipe. (Though we're not exactly gobbling it up by the gallon, there are ways to make it more palatable going down. Read on.) More important, semen is worth our scrutiny because, more than anything else, it is the barometer by which you can measure a guy's fertility and health. Hardy sperm semen-surf into a woman's vagina; off-color semen is a key indicator that something's physically amiss. Oh yes—and guys who enjoy spraying semen onto the bodies of their sexual partners need to cancel some of their subscriptions to XXX websites.

For such a fundamental part of the sexual experience, it's too bad that semen isn't a bit more seductive. After all, women separated from their beloved often hold on to a favorite shirt for a whiff of his scent, keep framed photos to gaze at him in the night, or perhaps engage in a bit of phone sex to hear the sultry rumble of his voice. But what woman in her right mind says to her boyfriend, "Here, honey. I know you're going away on business for two weeks, so would you mind ejaculating into this Dixie cup so I can taste your semen while you're away?" Not so much.

Yeah, it might look like watered-down Elmer's glue and taste like moist socks. But we've received plenty of questions about semen—perhaps because you've been keeping

SEMEN DOSSIER

Name: semen

Aliases: jizz, spunk, baby batter, cream, jism, hot milk, load, love juice, pearl jam, see, spoo, whipped cream, white honey, yogurt, oyster paste, wad

Characteristics: Smells like chlorine. Looks cloudy white. Tastes slightly sweet.

Vital stats: Made up of 65 percent fluid from the seminal vesicles, 30 to 35 percent from the prostate, and 5 percent from the vasa. Semen contains citric acid, free amino acids, fructose, enzymes, phosphorylcholine, prostaglandin, potassium, and zinc.

Hometown: prostate, by way of seminal vesicles

Last seen in testicles

your distance for too long. Time to hold your nose, ladies, and dive in!

Why does semen taste slightly sweet?

☞ Semen is sweet for the same reason breast milk is sweet—they're both designed to nourish living things. Nourishment means energy, and energy means sugar. In the case of semen, the sugar is fructose, a simple sugar similar to the blood sugar glucose. Fructose is the sweetest naturally occurring sugar, being about twice as sweet as table sugar (sucrose).

That sugar is nourishing the sperm, which constitute a mere 3 percent of the volume of any given ejaculation. They have their work cut out for them: They are only a few microns long and yet they have to swim their way through many centimeters of the female reproductive tract. That's a distance about 100,000 times their own length—more than equivalent to running a marathon. Since they can't "bulk up" with a big spaghetti meal the night before an ejaculation, where are they supposed to get the energy for this journey? From the semen, of course! Nature has arranged things so that sperm are literally swimming through food. And how do they eat? The fructose molecules are small enough to pass relatively easily through the "skin" (cell membrane) of the sperm.

If a guy's semen seems unusually sweet, that may be a bad sign. Overly sweet semen may be a symptom of diabetes. Diabetes, of course, can lead to a host of problems, not least of which is difficulty getting or keeping an erection.

Why is the consistency so . . . gooey?

☞ One of the more amazing qualities of semen is that it doesn't have a single consistency or viscosity. Just after ejaculation, normal semen is slightly sticky and jellylike. This is just perfect for keeping as much semen as possible at the back of the vagina, against the cervix, which is where the sperm need to go. If semen were as watery as, say, urine, most of it would drain quickly out of the vagina.

But sticky, jellylike semen is also harder for the sperm to swim through. So Nature has designed semen to slowly liquefy, which allows the sperm better access to the cervix and uterus. This liquefaction typically occurs about 15 minutes to 30 minutes after ejaculation—so at that point the semen will run out easily from a vagina. That's the guy's contribution to the infamous "wet spot" on the sheets. (Women contribute their own liquids, of course.)

If a guy's semen doesn't liquefy normally, that can contribute to infertility—and one of the tests done during a semen workup is a timing of liquefaction.

Sticky and gooey aren't so bad, actually. Most ladies have also spent time with salty, spunky, sour, and slimy. Why do some guys taste different from others?

☞ Many women know that all guys don't taste alike. As we just learned, semen is normally fairly sweet because it contains fructose. But the flavor of semen is affected by what a man eats or smokes. Generally speaking, semen should not taste bad—it shouldn't be bitter or have a strong odor. If it does, it could be because the guy is a smoker (of either cigarettes or marijuana), or because he's been drinking a lot of coffee or alcohol. Certain foods, such as asparagus and garlic, can give semen an off flavor because they contain high levels of certain enzymes.[33]

Also, semen can very in its saltiness. Semen is a mixture of two types of fluid: The stuff coming from the seminal vesicles is high in fructose, while the stuff coming from the prostate gland is slightly acidic and salty. If the seminal vesicles are blocked—which can occur in cases of male infertility—the semen will taste more salty than sweet. As men age, the contribution of the sweet seminal vesicle fluid can decline and, as the prostate grows larger, can leave semen tasting saltier. The same thing can happen if a man ejaculates frequently: The seminal vesicles don't have enough time to "reload" with sugary fluid; hence the semen, again, is saltier than normal. Whether a woman can detect such changes in salinity and, therefore, make inferences about her man's ejaculatory frequency is something that's not (yet) been explored scientifically.

Let's talk about quantity, not quality, for a moment. Does a man ejaculate more semen if he hasn't had sex in a long time?

☞ Yes, up to a point. The volume of a normal ejaculation is between 2 and 5 milliliters—5 milliliters being roughly equal to a teaspoon.[34] If a guy does not ejaculate for several days, the volume will increase slightly—perhaps by a couple of milliliters. That's why guys who are giving a

semen sample for medical reasons are asked not to ejaculate for two or three days.

Guys report that orgasms feel better if they abstain for
a couple of days, and one reason is probably the feel of
ejaculating a bigger "load."[35] It may take more contractions of the various muscles involved in ejaculation to
transport a larger-than-normal volume of semen, and it's
the contractions that are a large part of the pleasure of
orgasm.

But a man's semen capacity has definite limits. Once
the seminal vesicles and prostate gland are "full," production of the various fluids drops off and excess fluid is
simply reabsorbed. So unless your guy is a Taoist who is
practicing extreme ejaculatory control, there's no need
to abstain from ejaculations for more than a couple of
days or so.

Can a man ever ejaculate anything other than semen?

☞ Nope. As I mentioned earlier, guys frequently emit a
very small amount of pre-ejaculatory fluid when they're
having sex. (That's one of the reasons why the "withdrawal" method of contraception just doesn't work.) But
this fluid doesn't count because, of course, it's emitted
before ejaculation. The only other fluid that could possibly be expelled during ejaculation is urine, but that's not
physiologically possible (in a normal, healthy male); one
of the steps in the orgasmic cascade is the closure of the
tube that carries urine from the bladder. It's extremely
difficult (though not impossible) for a guy to urinate
while he has an erection, but it's impossible for him to
urinate during ejaculation.

If a guy doesn't ejaculate for a while, does he also get more horny?

☞ Since horniness is a function of testosterone, your question is really: Is there any connection between frequency of ejaculation and testosterone level? On the face of it, you might think Nature would design things so the answer was "yes." Guys who got increasingly horny the longer they didn't ejaculate would probably father more children than guys who didn't care whether they ejaculated or not. Research done in 2003 seems to support this, though the effect doesn't kick in as quickly as you might think. That study found that testosterone levels rose significantly after seven days of abstinence.[36]

You said earlier that larger testicles are a sign of fertility. Do larger testicles also mean more semen?

☞ Not quite. The larger the testicle, the more sperm. Testicles don't make the seminal fluids. They make the sperm that are added to those fluids like so many noodles to a pot of soup. If a guy is ejaculating unusually large loads, it's because he's got larger-than-normal seminal vesicles and a larger-than-normal prostate gland.

Well, then, how about this: the larger the penis, the farther the ejaculate flies?

☞ Nope. No correlation there either.

Hmm ... okay. So how far does a man ejaculate, assuming there isn't a vagina there to catch it? Maybe I've seen one too many drunken peeing contests.

☞ Depends on wind conditions. Seriously, there are no scientific data here. But there is an important point: Normally, semen is forcibly expelled from an erect penis—it "shoots," in other words. If it doesn't—if it just sort of dribbles out—that could be a sign of a clogged ejaculatory duct or some other problem, and it could impair a man's fertility.

How far the ejaculate actually shoots depends on whether the guy is helping the process with his hand or some other device that actively helps pump the semen out. If he pumps the shaft with the contraction, semen can fly farther. Under the right conditions, semen can easily be propelled several feet from the tip of the penis.

I know that some women are allergic to the latex in condoms, which makes sense. But what about women who swell up like inner tubes after unprotected sex? I've heard that some women are actually allergic to semen, and that's scary. Lots of us have painful sex—burning, itching, out-and-out pain. Sometimes it's just because we've engaged in particularly athletic sex. But what if it happens a lot, and an infection isn't to blame? Can semen really make us sick?

☞ Yes—and this is something a lot of women don't know about. While the prevalence of semen allergy is not known, the condition may be diagnosed in women who report symptoms that occur shortly after intercourse.[37] Symptoms may include itching, burning, and swelling in the genital area. In the most severe cases, hives or swelling may appear elsewhere on the body and the woman may experience difficulty breathing. Typically, symptoms occur within 30 minutes of intercourse, but in rare cases it may be hours or even days later. Semen

BURNING LOVE

Don't panic—just because you're experiencing symptoms, that doesn't necessarily mean you're allergic to semen. Bacterial vaginosis (BV) is the name of a condition in women in which the normal balance of bacteria in the vagina is disrupted, leading to an overgrowth of certain bacteria. It is sometimes accompanied by discharge, odor, pain, itching, or burning. BV is the most common vaginal infection in women of childbearing age. In the United States, as many as 16 percent of pregnant women have BV. Some activities or behaviors can upset the normal balance of bacteria in the vagina and put women at increased risk, including:

• Having a new sex partner or multiple sex partners

• Douching

• Using an intrauterine device (IUD) for contraception

Women with BV may have an abnormal vaginal discharge with an unpleasant odor. Some women report a strong fishlike odor, especially after intercourse. Discharge, if present, is usually white or gray; it can be thin. Women with BV may also have burning during urination or itching around the outside of the vagina, or both. Some women with BV report no signs or symptoms at all.

Source: www.cdc.gov/std/bv/STDFact-Bacterial-Vaginosis.htm

allergy is particularly suspected if symptoms go away with condom use or abstinence.

If you suspect you might be allergic to your partner's sperm, see a doctor. There are several techniques that can be tried to overcome the symptoms.

Time-out! This is awful—sort of like those kids you see on the Discovery Channel who live in bubbles because they're allergic to themselves. Semen allergies are right up there with unwanted pregnancies and cankles as things young women really do not want.

☞ It's okay—calm down. Allergies to semen are extremely rare. One "treatment option" is obviously abstinence. But more realistic options are using condoms, antihistamines, and, if the allergy is severe, desensitization, which is how allergists treat other kinds of allergies. If this is the case, where there are symptoms of swelling and pain, a visit to the gynecologist is also in order, as the woman may also have vaginitis (a vaginal infection) that is worsened by sexual contact. Irritation after sexual intercourse is more likely related to friction (caused by sex before appropriate lubrication), prolonged sex, or a preexisting vaginal infection.

Can guys be allergic to their own semen, too? Or, at least, not compatible with it?

☞ Yes, actually. In rare cases, men may create antibodies against their own sperm, and this is one of many reasons a guy may have impaired fertility.[38] An estimated one of every 10 men trying to conceive a child—roughly 2.5 million men in the United States alone—are either infertile or subfertile.[39] Another way to look at it is that in about 40 percent of infertile couples it's the man with the problem, in 40 percent it's the woman, and in 20 percent either both partners contribute or the cause is unknown. The main causes of male infertility are:

➡ Problems with the number, shape, or motility of sperm. Most commonly caused by varicoceles
➡ Problems with ejaculation
➡ Congenital absence of sperm
➡ Congenital malformations of the vas deferens or other reproductive structures
➡ Subclinical infections of the reproductive tract
➡ Sexually transmitted infections
➡ Hormonal abnormalities

What does a healthy sperm look like?

☞ Like a microscopic tadpole:

The head is where the genetic material is located—the "goods" that all the other parts are designed to propel to an egg. The acrosome is a layer of specialized

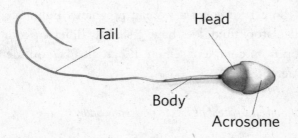

Sperm

molecules that can "dock" with the outer layer of an egg and begin the complicated process of transferring the male genes into the nucleus of the egg. The body and tail, as you can guess, are the "muscles" of the sperm and drive it forward with whiplike motions.

What's semen made of? And how, exactly, does it differ from pre-come? It all kind of looks the same.

☞ Like other bodily fluids, semen is mostly water. As we've seen, mixed into the water are ingredients such as sugar (fructose), vitamins, enzymes, minerals, calcium, and a range of proteins that give the semen its color, viscosity, and physical qualities. And, of course, it contains about 3 percent sperm cells. As a health food, it's not half bad—and it's only 36 calories per teaspoon!

Pre-ejaculatory fluid or "precome" is composed of somewhat mucus-like fluid from the prostate gland in which active sperm are usually observed. Typically, only a few drops of this fluid are emitted during the "plateau phase" of orgasm. This may be a matter of seconds or minutes prior to a full orgasm. From a functional standpoint, therefore, this fluid is the same as semen, because it can certainly get a woman pregnant! But since pre-ejaculatory fluid does have a slightly different composition from complete semen, it can also be considered a different fluid.

Can a man ejaculate if he has to pee really badly?

☞ Yes, he could, technically speaking—though if the urgency is really severe, it'll probably be distracting enough that he'll lose his erection. As I mentioned above, what's not possible (in a normal guy) is for him to pee if he wants to ejaculate really badly. As we've noted before, just prior to orgasm the tube leading to the bladder is squeezed shut so that semen can be propelled through the urethra and out of the penis. That means you can't pee and ejaculate at the same time. If that "valve" to the bladder is broken (as is common in some surgical procedures), then the semen goes "retrograde" and ends up in the bladder. The result is a "dry" ejaculation, which feels no different to the guy but certainly has some profound effects on his fertility!

Why do guys like to see themselves come? Is it pure vanity or is something else going on, like a desire for Ice-T's sex mirror as seen on Cribs?

☞ It's probably out of curiosity, at first. When guys hit puberty, the entire process of erection, orgasm, and ejaculation is intensely interesting. Even if you have read about all of it ahead of time, it's still amazing and not a little mysterious. So watching yourself come is kinda cool. How long it takes for the fascination to wear off depends on how easily bored the guy is.

This is one of my favorite questions from our lovely female forum: "Why do guys enjoy coming on women, whether it's the belly, breasts, or face? I've tried Neutrogena and I've tried semen—and I have to say, Neutrogena puts out the better moisturizer."

☞ First of all, it's just not true that all guys—or even most guys—like this kind of thing. Guys are not designed for this—Nature wants the guy inside when he ejaculates, not outside. And that's usually what feels best. The phenomenon of ejaculating outside of a woman may be a side effect of the classic "cum shot" in pornography—the thinking being that having the male actor withdraw at the crucial moment to show his ejaculation proves that he's not faking it. Or something. Guys (and women) watching such stuff may get the idea that this is normal or expected behavior, and thus do it even though some part of their brain is screaming at them to stop being such a dope and keep the damned thing inside, where it belongs.

Is there a correlation between ejaculation (amount and distance) and virility?

☞ Men with low ejaculate volume may have a low testosterone level or a blockage of the ejaculatory ducts. The most common way to tell that there's a problem is if the sperm drips or dribbles out rather than spurting out. Also, if the sperm keeps leaking out of the penis for a few minutes after intercourse has finished, that could indicate that a blockage is present. And if, during or after ejaculation, the man feels pain anywhere, particularly in the groin, that indicates a problem. If there is blood in the ejaculate, seek medical advice. All of these symptoms can indicate a problem with either testosterone levels or a blockage that can result in infertility.

Do men ejaculate more semen with more foreplay?

☞ Some men report that to be true, but we have no data on this. For many men, more foreplay results in a better orgasm, and many men equate that with increased fluid. What's probably happening, however, is that they are experiencing a couple more of the pulsing muscle spasms that accompany an orgasm (in both males and females), whether or not those spasms are carrying semen.

Does clearer semen mean anything—like purer semen?

☞ Absolutely! But it's not what you think. Clear semen may actually mean a guy is shooting blanks. Remember that sperm makes up only 3 percent of the ejaculate. It's the sperm that makes the semen cloudy. Men who have a vasectomy tend to have clear semen after it liquefies— which happens about 30 minutes after ejaculation.

Surely not every ejaculation is pearly white and rife with sperm. This may sound gross, but what about pink semen or yellowish semen? Semen that looks like it would fit right in at a Phish show?

☞ Pink or red-tinged semen is the result of blood mixing with the semen, either in the prostate or during ejaculation. This can mean a number of things, most of which require attention but which are not life-threatening. In most cases, the guy has a bacterial infection of some type or an enlarged prostate. Rarely is it prostate cancer. The only way to find out is to have him go to a urologist for a complete workup. Bottom line: Pink may look cute in a shirt or a tie, but it's definitely not cool in semen.

Semen that is yellow or greenish in color is a sign of infection, often due to gonorrhea. If it is gonorrhea, treatment is simple with the use of antibiotics.

One of our readers would like me to ask if semen is good for her hair, like olive oil.

☞ Who makes this stuff up? Would you put maple syrup in your hair? I don't think so. Quite aside from the fact that you'd need more than a couple of guys to ejaculate on your head in order to "shampoo" with semen, there is nothing in semen that would either clean or nourish your hair.

HARD FACTS ABOUT SEMEN

Bands named after semen: 10cc, Lovin' Spoonful, Pearl Jam

Nutritional properties of semen: a carbohydrate fluid with about 36 calories per teaspoon

Percentage of guys who've tasted their own semen: Who would admit to that?

LET'S TALK ABOUT SEX, BABY

The Ins and Outs of Intercourse

Clinton lied. A man might forget where he parks or where he lives, but he never forgets oral sex, no matter how bad it is.

—Former First Lady Barbara Bush

AH, SEX. IT LEADS men to war; it leads women to kill; it leads politicians to lie. It sells everything from jeans to golf clubs. It's spawned more fights than religion and more regrettable hookups than cheap tequila. And if it weren't for sex, none of us would be here. Our Neanderthal forebears engaged in sex for procreation; it's a natural instinct to sustain survival of the species. But somewhere along the way, we discovered that sex is also pleasurable. Trying to conceive is just one teensy little reason that many of us lock loins. Other motivators include revenge, guilt, too much beer, and sometimes even love. As sex has become more and more important, it's turned into a commodity like anything else: We want the fastest cars, the biggest houses, the tallest heels, and, goddamn it, the best sex, too. Women

95

have been taught to know their bodies, to take control of their orgasms, to demand nothing less than fireworks and bliss.

Good for us! But while we've done a terrific job of figuring out how to please ourselves (and how to fake orgasms or buy vibrators, when necessary), how many times have you thought to yourself, *Gee. I wonder how my husband/boyfriend/hunky masseuse feels when he's about to ejaculate? Where's he feeling his orgasm? How was it for him?* Not so much, right? That's because we take it as gospel that guys are naturally having a fantastic time in bed. They always get to have an orgasm; erections are usually easy to come by; and they're almost always up for action. Women are more mysterious creatures. We need coaxing, romance, candlelight. You might know that, in order to achieve orgasm, you must be splayed across the bed at a 60-degree angle with a pillow between your knees eating an apple while "Groove Is in the Heart" plays on a loop. Congratulations! "Know thyself," Socrates famously said. But if he were sexually active in the twenty-first century, he might have added: "Know your sexual partner." If you want to have the best possible sex, it's just as important you have a handle on what's going on with him as with yourself. So put down the vibrator and get reading! (And get some better taste in music!)

I think I can speak for most women when I say that men seem to climax a lot more easily than women. How long does a guy typically pound away before he reaches orgasm?

☞ Studies in which couples were actually observed having sex or in which one partner timed sex with a stop-

watch (as opposed to surveys in which pe
asked how long they have sex) show a wide
the length of lovemaking, ranging from abo
utes to 40 or more minutes. The average? About 7.5
minutes in one of the more recent studies.[40] That's
longer (believe it or not) than in studies done decades
ago. In the discussion of marital sex in his classic book
about male sexuality, researcher Alfred Kinsey specu-
lated that for perhaps three-fourths of all males, orgasm was reached within 2 minutes of initiation of
coitus, and that this was "a frequent source of marital
conflict."[41]

Although this 2-minute average time to male orgasm
probably sounds damned short, it's actually rather
leisurely compared to our closest primate relatives:
Chimpanzee sex lasts an average of 8 seconds, and go-
rilla sex lasts an average of a minute.[42] The reason for
that brevity is clear: Animals are rather vulnerable when
they're having sex, so there's a premium put on a wham-
bam-thank-you-ma'am approach to things. But just because fast sex is in Nature's best interest doesn't mean it's
the ideal. Far from it. Volumes have been written on the
desirability of prolonging sex so that it is more generally
enjoyable and so that the woman has a more realistic
chance for achieving an orgasm (women, in general,
taking longer to reach orgasm than men even with direct clitoral stimulation).

There are entire schools of "sexology" that advocate
delayed male orgasm. The Taoist approach to sex, which
has been popularized in this country by Jolan Chang, is a
very female-oriented approach to lovemaking. Various

techniques are suggested for slowing down the male sexual response and postponing male orgasm. Indeed, Chang advocates an approach to sex that deemphasizes male orgasm. Men can—and should—have sex without orgasm, he suggests.[43] Not only does this allow a man to make love for as long as he wants with a firm erection, but it creates many more opportunities for variation in position and satisfaction of the woman's sexual desires.

That sounds great and all, but what if you're not dating a Taoist and your partner is usually ready to orgasm before you've even turned down the TV? How can we slow things down a bit without making the guy feel bad about his sexual technique?

☞ There are several methods you could try. One is the "start and stop" approach: As soon as the guy feels like he's getting close to ejaculating, he stops thrusting and either holds his penis still in the vagina or withdraws until the feeling (but not the erection) fades. Some people use the "squeeze technique," in which the guy withdraws his penis and either he or his partner gently squeezes the penis right below the head (glans) for a few seconds. The Tao folks recommend a "pressure" technique that is less cumbersome than the "squeeze" approach. They suggest that when a guy feels ejaculation is near, he use a finger or two to apply pressure to his own perineum—that's the area between the anus and testicles. He can slow or stop his thrusting at the same time, but he needn't withdraw completely. Finally, you might experiment with different sexual positions. Some guys find some positions particularly erotic, which makes it more difficult for them to control their ejaculation. Avoiding those positions (or reserving them for "dessert") might help slow things down a bit.

How about frequency of sex? Sex is everywhere in the media—from TV shows to movies to marketing campaigns. There is a reason The Forty-Year-Old Virgin *is so funny. I mean, unless you're a priest, how on earth could you reach middle age without having done it? My friends and I aren't having constant sex, either. But you'd think it's normal for people to have sex every day—at least! But that can't be right. Can it? (Gulp. Sob.)*

☞ So much depends on the circumstances! Certainly for a young couple in the early throes of a love relationship, it's perfectly normal that they have a lot of sex—daily if not more frequently. But as most people know from experience, this phase of a sexual relationship hardly ever continues for more than a few months at that initially fiery tempo. What's "normal" in a long-term relationship varies with the age of the couple and the age of the relationship—and, not surprisingly, the frequency of sex declines with both.

As for averages, it's hard to find good data because so many surveys are biased in one way or another. Online surveys, for example, are clearly biased toward younger and more affluent respondents. One of the most careful studies done in recent years is the American Sexual Behavior Study from 2006. Here's what the study authors found.

FREQUENCY OF SEXUAL INTERCOURSE

(mean number per year)

Married couples

Age	Frequency of intercourse
18–29	109.1
30–39	87.0
40–49	70.2
50–59	52.5
60–69	32.2
70+	17.2

Unmarried couples

Age	Frequency of intercourse
18–29	73.4
30–39	67.8
40–49	48.2
50–59	29.3
60–69	16.2
70+	3.3

So you can see that even young married couples are having sex, on average, about once every three days or so, and the frequency goes down from there. What really matters, of course, is not whether you are having more or less sex than "normal" but whether the sex you have is satisfying. Some couples can be quite content with very little sex, while others desire much more.

Let's say one or both partners isn't sexually satisfied within the relationship. What about "extracurricular sex"? Guys get a bad rap as being the major cheaters in relationships, but I know plenty of women who've been the ones to look elsewhere once things got a little bit slow. Are there any facts here?

☞ Again, data are often suspect because of "responder bias." Quite high levels of adultery have been reported in the past—as high as 70 percent of married women, for example, in Shere Hite's infamous report. Even Alfred Kinsey and his colleagues found that half of all married men had an affair at some point in their marriage, and that 26 percent of married women had had extramarital sex by their forties.

But the more scientifically rigorous, and current, study mentioned earlier finds lower (though still significant) levels of adultery. The best estimates are that about 3–4 percent of currently married people have a sexual partner besides their spouse in a given year and

ORAL SEX

Here's what Alfred Kinsey and his colleagues found out when they asked men and women about their experiences with oral sex:

Percentage of males who said they had performed cunnilingus:
    before marriage, about 10%
    in marriage, 48.9%

Percentage of females who said they had performed fellatio:
    before marriage, 19.1%
    in marriage, 45.5%

about 15–18 percent of ever-married people have had a sexual partner other than their spouse while married.[44]

Let's talk about women's sexual desires for a minute. Blow jobs are pretty far down on the list — I have yet to meet the woman who enjoys burying her head in a guy's dank, pheromone-laced pubes for what seems like an eternity, arranging her lips to simulate a toothless vagina, while either choking or wheezing in the process. But men love blow jobs so much that we keep giving 'em out anyway. What do men love so much about that experience, as opposed to actual sex?

☞ Men love it probably because it feels good and it's a different type of sensation from that of vaginal intercourse. Many women enjoy oral sex for the same reason. Variety is the spice of life and all that. Of course, there may be other reasons as well. Some guys (such as Bill Clinton) don't think fellatio counts as "having sex" and so they may want this kind of stimulation to ease their guilty consciences. Some guys — and maybe some women, too — may think of fellatio as "naughty" or "bad" and experience a heightened stimulation from the feelings of engaging in something illicitly erotic. It's also possible that some guys view fellatio as a power trip — they get off on the notion that fellatio is a submissive act and they like the feeling of domination it gives them. (Of course, fellatio isn't inherently a submissive act — it's simply oral sex. Whether it's given freely and lovingly or hesitantly and under coercion is entirely a matter of the people involved.)

What's weirder still is that many guys seem to love watching us as we're giving the blow job. What's so exciting about a head bobbing up and down?

☞ Humans—and especially men—are intensely visual creatures. Of all the sensory receptors in the body, 70 percent are in the eyes.[45] And a massive portion of our brains is devoted to processing visual information. In other words, we like to watch. We are easily aroused by sexual imagery of all kinds. And that includes watching ourselves and our partners during sex.

However, men may be more avid in their desire for visual stimulation than women. In a revealing statistic, Alfred Kinsey and his colleagues found that 40 percent of the males in their studies preferred to have sexual activities in some light, compared with only 19 percent of the females.[46] In addition, men make up two-thirds of users of sexually explicit Internet sites and account for 77 percent of online time.[47]

A friend who wishes to remain anonymous asks this question: What happens in a guy's body when he comes, and does it feel the same as a woman's orgasm? I'm sure all women can relate to this: We're giving a guy a blow job, and suddenly he stiffens, shudders, and shoves our head onto his penis with brute force. Is it the same feelings causing that response as the ones we feel when we climax?

☞ For all their differences, men and women's sexual responses are remarkably similar, and in all likelihood their orgasms have the same diversity of intensities and degrees of pleasure. In their classic book on human sexuality, Masters and Johnson noted that "aside from obvious anatomic variants, men and women are homogenous in their physiologic responses to sexual stimuli."[48] This isn't surprising, since the male and female genitalia are built from the same parts. In fact, a male's genitalia are indistinguishable from a female's for the first two months of fetal development.[49] All the basic patterns of cells, nerves, and blood vessels are laid down then. Only when a fetal boy's body gets flooded with testosterone does his penis begin to form (from clitoral tissue), his testicles develop (from tissues destined for the labia and ovaries), and internal organs such as the prostate and seminal vesicles form.

All of this means that a guy's genitals and body respond to sexual stimulation in very similar ways to women's. One of the first ways is that the arteries feeding the penis relax and open up. (The same thing happens to the clitoris and, to a lesser extent, a woman's breasts.) A guy's testicles will tighten and come closer to his body as sexual excitement builds. Before ejaculation can occur, the prostate, seminal vesicles, and vas deferens contract rhythmically. A "valve" leading to the bladder closes so that semen can't be forced backwards. These contractions and the buildup of seminal fluids in the upper part of the urethra produce a feeling that orgasm is inevitable. This feeling lasts between 2 and 3 seconds and then the entire sexual machinery, including the muscles in the penis and around the anus, contracts in unison in intervals a little faster than one a second (0.8 seconds, to be exact). You'll see spurts of semen expelled during these contractions. Two or three of the spurts propel the bulk of the semen from the penis. After that, contractions may continue with less expulsive force and on a more irregular rhythm for another two to four cycles.

The rhythms of muscle contractions in the female genitalia during orgasm have exactly the same pattern and timing. The major difference between the sexes is that following ejaculation men experience a latency period in which further erection and orgasm are not possible, whereas women can immediately begin "ramping up" to another orgasm.

The fact that orgasms feel as wonderful to women as to men has been supported by several types of studies.[50] In one, college students provided descriptions of their orgasms. Researchers compared the descriptions using a standard psychological rating scale, and there were no distinguishable differences between men's and women's descriptions. Both males and females tended to describe orgasm with words such as "waves of pleasure in my body," corresponding to the rhythmic muscle contractions that occur during orgasm. In another study, 70 expert judges could not reliably differentiate between descriptions of orgasms by men and by women.

Another one from the peanut gallery: Women can feel pain during sex for a variety of reasons, from lack of lubrication to more serious issues like the painful spasms of vaginismus. Do men ever find sex painful, and if so, why?

☞ Yes, sex can be painful for a guy. There are a number of reasons for this unfortunate circumstance. Peyronie's disease, which is a severe curvature in an erect penis, can cause painful bending of the penis during sex. Some guys who are uncircumcised have a foreskin that is "stuck" over the head of the penis. This condition, called phimosis, can make sex quite painful indeed for the guy. A relatively common infection of the testicles called epididymitis can make the testicles so sensitive that the motions of sex become painful. If a guy has an obstruction of his ejaculatory ducts, he may experience a pain or ache in the area of his prostate when he ejaculates. And the sores associated with some STIs (such as herpes lesions) can also make sex a rather masochistic act for a guy.

What happens if a guy doesn't have an orgasm—is there any limit to how long an erection can last if it just doesn't happen? Eventually, he just must want to pack it in and go home, right?

☞ Maintaining an erection without ejaculating is certainly possible, and advocates of delayed ejaculation report that this state can be maintained for more than two hours with practice.[51] But erections much longer than this are actually dangerous. Because an erection is caused by blood that is trapped in the penis, the oxygen levels in the penile tissue can become dangerously low if the erection doesn't end. In these situations, men complain of severe pain with the prolonged erection. Such an undesired and prolonged erection, called priapism, is actually a medical emergency. Without prompt attention, irreversible damage can set in (yuck) and complete impotence can result (major yuck).

If a guy masturbates before sex, will he have more stamina?

☞ You bet. The entire sexual-response cycle will slow down after an ejaculation and latency period. This is actually a rather common "technique" for young men who don't want to ejaculate the second they enter a woman—or even before they enter a woman! But this

ASK A GUY

Can my husband tell if I'm faking it?

A 35-year-old male replies:
Sometimes my wife just wants me to finish, so she'll start moaning louder and talking dirty to me. I can tell she's faking it, but it doesn't matter. It turns me on and always makes me come faster.

kind of "pump priming" can get dicey for older guys or guys who aren't naturally so quick on the draw. Masturbating prior to sex can very easily lead to an outright erectile failure and can make orgasm nigh on impossible—which rather defeats the purpose.

If a man works out a lot, does that mean he'll have good stamina in bed?

☞ There's an old saying in the field of urology: "What's good for the heart is good for the penis." That means that things like losing weight, eating a healthy diet, and exercise will all help a guy maintain his sexual prowess. As a general rule, healthy, fit guys will have a more reliable and robust sexual response. Of course, that may not mean they have more "stamina." In younger guys, it may mean they're apt to ejaculate faster than a sedentary guy who smokes and drinks a lot, at least in the first orgasm of the night.

Can a man orgasm without ejaculating?

☞ Yes—and the reverse can happen, too: Guys can ejaculate without orgasm.

Although they usually happen at the same time, ejaculation and the pleasurable feelings of orgasm are separate physiological events. And although they are designed to occur simultaneously, they can occur separately under certain conditions.

For example, some types of prostate surgery unavoidably damage the "valve" that normally closes off the bladder during ejaculation. Men who have had such surgery, therefore, have "dry" orgasms—the semen is expelled in a "retrograde" direction into the bladder. These men have orgasms (which feel perfectly normal) but no outward ejaculation.

The flip side of this equation is also possible, albeit with technological assistance. Men can be "forced" to ejaculate without an accompanying orgasm by applying electrical stimulation to the proper nerves at the base of the spine. This technique can be used to obtain sperm from men with spinal cord injuries for use in artificial insemination or in vitro fertilization. In the absence of artificial stimulation or damage caused by surgery or illness, however, when there's orgasm, there's ejaculation.

Do men ever fake orgasms, the way women do, just to get things over with?

☞ If a guy has a condition that prevents him from ejaculating normally (such as the prostate surgery patients just mentioned), then theoretically he can fake an orgasm as easily as a woman can fake hers. It just requires good acting abilities. But for the vast majority of guys, orgasm equals ejaculation. So if a guy is grunting like a bull and claims to be coming but you don't see (or sense) any semen, then he hasn't had an orgasm and for some perverse reason is trying to fool you into thinking he did.

Women have different types of orgasms. There's the more common clitoral orgasm, and then there's the Holy Grail of Sexual Pleasure— the superintense vaginal one, which some ladies only dream about. Does a man orgasm only from his penis?

☞ As explained earlier, male orgasm and ejaculation involve muscular contractions of the penis, anus, prostate gland, testicles, seminal vesicles, and vas deferens. It's a whole party of muscles and body parts, in other words, not just a penile affair. So, no—a guy doesn't orgasm just with his penis.

Why do guys seem to be so sleepy after orgasm?

☞ Let's see. . . . Most people have sex in bed. At the end of the day. With the lights out or turned down low. In this setting and situation, it would be awfully unusual if men didn't fall asleep after sex—in fact, you'll probably notice that they fall asleep whether they have sex or not. On the other hand, watch a guy who's just made love to you in the middle of the day in some "clandestine" location such as a park, the office, or the car. Bet he's not falling asleep!

So the answer is probably that the cliché of the guy snoring seconds after having sex has less to do with the sex and more to do with his general fatigue.

Having said that, there are some physiological changes that accompany orgasm that promote a relaxed, satisfied feeling and that could certainly promote slumber. After a man or a woman has an orgasm, a bunch of different hormones and compounds are released, including oxytocin, prolactin, gamma-aminobutyric acid, and endorphins. The hormone oxytocin has been associated with maternal bonding with infants and with a tendency to nuzzle and cuddle.

So given all this, don't feel too bad if a guy isn't in a hugely talkative or energetic mood after sex.

On the other hand, some men are anything but sleepy afterward— and during sex! Why do guys who are buttoned-down accountants in real life scream things like "Mommy!" and "You like that, bitch!" when in the throes of passion? Is this a window into the psyche?

☞ I'm not sure about that "Mommy" bit. That might suggest some kind of developmental regression going on. But "potty mouth" coming from an otherwise mild-mannered guy isn't that uncommon. Sex is primal. It engages very ancient parts of our brains—parts that evolved millions of years before the thinking, analyzing, socially conscious parts. When guys have sex, they grunt, they moan, they almost growl. It's a short step from those primal vocalizations to other highly charged, deeply sexual, or otherwise offensive words and phrases such as "fuck," "fuck me," "cunt," "bitch," "slut," "whore," and so on. These types of words may even be stored in a different area of the brain. Some people with very specific brain lesions caused by strokes completely lose their ability to speak, except that they can still swear a blue streak. This can be frightening to family members, but it's not uncommon and suggests that "swearwords" are stored in other, deeper, parts of the brain than the rest of our language abilities. Perhaps they are stored, or at least are associated, with the same reptilian brain regions that govern our lust and are thus activated and more readily vocalized during sex.

Here's a great question that's come up time and again with my friends: Is there such a thing as equipment compatibility—or noncompatibility? You know, a penis that just can't fit in a vagina no matter how much chemistry exists out of bed?

☞ Yes. There are ranges in sizes of both penises and vaginas, and some fits are better than others. If the penis is relatively too big for a small vagina, you'll get equipment noncompatibility. The penis may be a perfectly normal size, but if the vagina is small, it will hurt. This is common as women age and a condition called atrophic vaginitis occurs. In this condition, the lack of estrogen actually makes the vagina less elastic and therefore essentially "smaller." In this case, it can help to increase the lubricants. In general, however, most vaginas are very accommodating, especially when the woman is turned on, and most can handle all sizes—but only when lubricated! I can't stress enough that, if foreplay is too short and the lubrication is not there, the vagina will not accommodate a penis of any size without pain.

How about store-bought lubrication? Surely that will help things along, no?

☞ There are lots of reasons a woman might not produce enough natural lubrication to make sex the easy, pleasurable thing it's supposed to be. After menopause, for example, the vagina naturally makes less lubricant during arousal. Of course, if a woman isn't "wet," it may also be that the guy's in too much of a hurry and hasn't engaged in enough foreplay. Whatever the reason, if a woman isn't producing enough natural lubrication, augmenting things with some other type will make everything go better for both partners. Just remember a few things: Don't use an oil-based lubricant such as petroleum jelly, butter, or baby oil if your partner is using a latex condom—the oil will weaken the condom and increase the chances it will leak. Water-

DR. FISCH'S SEX SMOOTHIE

Here's a really easy and tasty way to enhance your sexuality by adding natural vitamins and antioxidants to your diet. The recipe below is for a single serving. Just multiply if you want to make more.

Ingredients

$1/2$ cup 100% pomegranate juice

$1/2$ cup yogurt (can be plain or vanilla, fat-free or reduced-fat)

$1/2$ a ripe banana (you can substitute an equivalent amount of any other fruit that you like, such as raspberries, strawberries, blackberries, blueberries, peaches, mango—you name it!)

Add the ingredients to a blender, whirl for 30 seconds or so, and enjoy!

based lubricants such as K-Y Jelly or Astrog
just as well and don't harm condoms. And
trying to get pregnant, take the time to bec
cated naturally, because any additional lubr_____,
use may interfere with the sperm's ability to swim up
into your uterus. Finally, if you're thinking about anal
sex, follow the adage "Too much lubricant is just
enough."

Okay. Add lubricant to the shopping list. Got it. Anything else our readers should pick up from the store — or avoid — before sex?

☞ The first thing to think about is what not to drink or eat. Alcohol is the biggest killer of good sex that I know. A glass of wine to relax a little? Probably fine. But it's really, really easy to keep drinking after that, and the more you drink, the harder it's going to be for the guy to get an erection and for the woman to get an orgasm. Instead of alcohol, I suggest drinking something healthy, such as fruit juice, water into which you add fresh lemon slices, or my Sex Smoothie (see box).

I always knew you were a smoothie, Harry. Anyway, how about what a guy eats? Is there any link between food and sexual performance?

☞ Absolutely! This is a big topic, of course. I'm going to focus here on a few of the key food nutrients that have a clear link to sexual performance.

First are foods that promote the production of a chemical in the body called nitric oxide. This is actually a gas that is released in minute amounts and is vital to both healthy blood vessels and the ability to get an erection.

FOOD SOURCES FOR BIOFLAVONOIDS

Bioflavonoids	Food sources
Anthocyanidins	Berries, cherries, grapes, fruit skins, and true fruit juices
Catechins	True teas (not herbal teas)
Flavanones	Citrus
Flavones	Grains, celery, parsley, and other herbs
Flavonols	Grapefruit, oranges, apple skin, berries, onions, endive, radishes, tomatoes, leeks, broccoli, and red wine

Nitric oxide is made from an amino acid called arginine. The following foods are rich in arginine:

- Beans
- Walnuts
- Cold-water fish such as salmon and tuna
- Soy products
- Oats
- Almonds

Another class of nutrients important for sexual health are the bioflavonoids. These are plant compounds that work like antioxidants, scavenging by-products of the body's metabolism or harmful molecules resulting from exposure to environmental pollutants like smog, cigarette smoke, or pesticides. Fruits and vegetables are the main sources of bioflavonoids. The table shows the types of bioflavonoids and some of the best food sources for each.

What's the buzz with pomegranate juice? It seems like the latest cure for what ails you—including a drooping sex drive.

☞ Pomegranate juice is great stuff. Expensive, but great. It's packed with vitamins and natural antioxidants. Although, as mentioned before, taking additional antioxidants in the form of megadoses of vitamins or supplements hasn't been shown to increase fertility, keeping natural sources of antioxidants (such as blueberries, broccoli, and a host of other fruits and vegetables) in our diet is probably what Nature intends. Research from several quarters suggests that natural antioxidants are "heart healthy" and may reduce the buildup of plaques that could clog arteries. As I've said repeatedly, what's good for the heart is good for the penis, so having a glass of pomegranate juice every day is probably a good thing.

Okay, okay. Pomegranate juice is a good way to get some antioxidants. Never mind that it costs five bucks at Whole Foods—it's worth it! What about other sources—in foods, for example?

☞ Lots of foods contain antioxidants, and they'll all help a guy's sexual health. As you'll see, many of these foods also contain the other nutrients we've been talking about. The general message is obvious: Fresh, whole foods are always going to be better for you than refined or processed foods. Here are some of the best foods for upping your antioxidant levels:[52]

- ➡ Berries
- ➡ Walnuts
- ➡ Sunflower seeds
- ➡ Pomegranates
- ➡ Ginger
- ➡ Citrus fruits
- ➡ Beans

- ➡ Kale
- ➡ Red cabbage
- ➡ Artichoke
- ➡ Brussels sprouts
- ➡ Spinach
- ➡ Garlic

Will taking vitamins help a guy's sex drive and stamina?

☞ Anything that adds to a guy's overall health is going to help his sex drive and stamina. Most often this involves subtracting things from his diet: the doughnuts, cookies, sweets, chips, french fries, fast food, and overprocessed foods of all types. No need to be fascist about it, of course. A few beers and some chips on the weekend? Fine. But every day? Not if he wants peak sexual performance. This isn't the place for a treatise on healthy eating, so I'll just remind you of something I mentioned before: The real dietary evils are sugar and refined carbohydrates, because these "foods" throw the body's insulin response out of whack, which leads to rapid conversion of the carbs to fat, increased hunger, and a lack of necessary vitamins and minerals.

To answer your question: Yes, a standard (nonmegadose) multivitamin tablet each day will help keep your body healthy. The table facing lists the daily recommended levels of vitamins and minerals for men from the 2006 *Essential Guide to Nutrient Requirements* of the Institute of Medicine.

DAILY RECOMMENDED LEVELS OF VITAMINS AND MINERALS FOR MEN

Vitamins

- A—900 mcg (or ~3,000 IU)

- B_6—1.3 mg

- B_{12}—2.4 mcg

- C—90 mg

- D—5 mcg

- E—15 mg (or ~24 IU)

- Folate (sometimes listed as vitamin B_9)— 400 mcg

- Thiamin—1.2 mg

- Riboflavin—1.3 mg

- Niacin—35 mg

- Biotin—30 mg

- Pantothenic acid—5 mg

Minerals

- Calcium—1,000 mg

- Magnesium—400 mg

- Selenium—55 micrograms

- Zinc—11 mg

Is there really such thing as an aphrodisiac?

☞ Yes and no. Ever hear of the placebo effect? That's when an inert substance or procedure produces real results because of the strong belief of the person taking the substance or submitting to the procedure. The placebo effect works—it is demonstrated practically every week in scientific studies of drug effectiveness. People will report being relieved of their depression or anxiety, for example, even though they've been taking a sugar pill. So if a man eats oysters and believes they're going to make him a real stud, there's every chance that he'll "perform" differently. In that sense—and that sense only—aphrodisiacs work. The list of alleged aphrodisiacs is very long, of course, and includes things such as powdered rhinoceros horn, dried tiger penis, and the crushed shells of certain beetles (aka "Spanish fly"). None of these has been proven to have any independent effect on sexual desire or ability—aside from the placebo effect, that is.

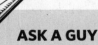

ASK A GUY

How do different positions feel different for a guy?

I think a lot of guys like doggie-style because it puts pressure and friction on the underside of the penis rather than on the top, and that feels better. It's also easy not to have the pressure of your girlfriend staring at you sometimes. The face-to-face sometimes can cause performance anxiety.

HARD FACTS ABOUT INTERCOURSE

Percentage of the male population who engage only in man-on-top (missionary position) sex: 70

Speed of a typical ejaculate: 28 miles per hour

Speed of Daisuke Matsuzaka fast ball: 90-plus miles per hour

Percentage of men who have not had vaginal sex by age 19: 11

Percentage of women who have not had vaginal sex by age 19: 9

Percentage of women who have faked an orgasm: 48

Percentage of men who prefer to have sex with some amount of light on: 40

Percentage of women who prefer light during sex: 19

Percentage of women who say they've never had an orgasm during intercourse: 25

The three countries where people lose their virginity at the earliest ages: Iceland (15.6 years old); Germany (15.9); Sweden (16.1)

The three countries where people lose their virginity the latest: India (19.8); Vietnam (19.6); Indonesia (19.1)

SINK OR SWIM

The Delicate Sciences of Contraception and Birth Control

REMEMBER WHEN *SEX AND the City*'s Miranda Hobbes got pregnant with her sometimes boyfriend, Steve? She had lazy ovaries, and he was operating with only one ball after having a testicle removed. Still, they managed to get knocked up—and, as Miranda sobbed, "win the Special Olympics of contraception." Meanwhile, baby-crazed Charlotte York MacDougal and her husband, Trey, whose plumbing was in perfect working order, realized that even trust funds and high-thread-count sheets didn't matter when it came to procreation. Kind of scary, isn't it? You can plan, hope, pray, sleep with a pristine copy of *What to Expect When You're Expecting* under your pillow, and have sex five times per day . . . and still not get pregnant. Scarier still, you can have a drunken (yet protected) tryst with your uniballed ex-boyfriend and end up with a Babies "R" Us registry. The seemingly arbitrary fertility gods have sent countless women harboring baby lust scurrying to a fertility specialist. Actually, though, the process is less random than you might fear, so don't toss out the Ortho Tri-Cyclen just yet.

Women know that eggs have an approximately 28-day cycle, and we get a nice little reminder of this every month just in case we forget. But what about sperm? What's their life span?

☞ What you're probably interested in is how long sperm live once they're ejaculated. I'll get to that in a second, but since you asked about "life span" I'll give you the full answer. Given that a healthy guy will make several hundred million sperm every day, you might think making the little fellas would be simple. Hardly. It actually takes between two and three months to make a fully functioning sperm. They begin as ordinary-looking body cells—featureless and roughly spherical. Over the course of weeks, the cell divides so that the resulting sperm will carry only half of the normal complement of chromosomes (so that when it unites with the egg, the resulting embryo will have the normal 46). It also grows a tail and transforms into the tadpole-like swimmer you learned about in high school biology class. The sperm migrate through increasingly larger tubes that all finally converge on the large-bore tubes called the vas deferens. The live, ready-for-action sperm are stored in the somewhat enlarged terminal ends of the vas deferens just before they enter the prostate.

Now to your real question. Once they are ejaculated, the sperm can live anywhere from a few minutes to nine days. It all depends on the conditions in which they find themselves postorgasm. If the semen is simply expelled into the world (i.e., a tissue, the floor, or a toilet), the little guys perish within minutes. But if they're lucky enough to end up at the back of a comfy vagina, they can live anywhere from two to nine days.[53] Turns out that some women's reproductive tracts are more chemically welcoming to sperm than others. The acid level of some vaginal secretions and cervical mucus is so high that they are actually toxic to sperm and may be the cause of infertility. Often this is the result of a low-grade bacterial infection, which can usually be cleared up with a course of an appropriate antibiotic.[54]

So the nine-day sperm are obviously more desirable than the two-day, at least in terms of fertility. Are they more likely to stick around if the guy is younger? Or do sperm improve with age, like fine wine, and become more durable?

☞ As with most things having to do with raw fertility (as opposed to, say, skill in lovemaking), younger is better. Every aspect of semen quality—not just the ability of the sperm to swim—declines slowly with age.[55] The volume of semen ejaculated declines with age. And the proportion of sperm that are abnormally shaped increases with time.

Of course, we're talking averages here. Men age at different rates. Some chronologically young guys will actually be biologically "old" and infertile, while some

"old men" will be perfectly able to keep on fathering
children.

*What about the whole "boxers versus briefs" thing? I've heard
rumors that guys shouldn't wear tightie whities because they restrict sperm production (and they look kind of silly on guys over age
12 or so).*

☞ It's true that the choice of boxers or briefs is a tad more
complicated than most guys realize. Nature designed the
testicles to hang in the breeze, because the machinery
that makes sperm cells works best in temperatures several degrees below body temperature. Warming the testicles in any way—by sitting in a hot tub or working for
long periods with a warm laptop computer—will impair
a guy's fertility to some extent.

Boxer underwear (or no underwear at all) lets the
testicles hang more or less as Nature intended. Briefs
don't—and so, yes, tight underwear can be too tight, for
fertility if nothing else. Some scientists have actually
done experiments that demonstrate this. David Karabinus, who studies animal fertility at the University of
Arizona, wrapped bull's testes in cloth (that must have
been a dicey bit of methodology!) and found that sperm
quality dropped considerably.[56] Ron Weber and colleagues in the Netherlands measured the temperature of
the testicles of guys wearing boxers and compared them
with that of the tightie-whitie boys. As expected, the
boxer crowd was cooler—literally.

Of course, we're talking about relatively small differences. If wearing briefs made guys permanently sterile,
you can bet that that fashion would become extinct

faster than you can say "hypogonadism." But the effect is at least somewhat there in the short term, so if you and a guy want to make a baby, suggest he switch to boxers or simply go "commando" (meaning dispensing with the entire business of underwear).

So assuming the guy's wearing underwear (I'm sure my husband will be delighted to know that it's best for him to let his testicles flow freely in the breeze!), what about when it comes off? What's the best position to be in to get pregnant? One enterprising woman in my yoga class swears by hanging upside down after sex in order to force the sperm to trickle in the right direction.

☞ There aren't any scientific studies that I know of regarding the best sexual positions for baby-making, but the missionary (man on top) position is typically considered optimal for conception. The idea is simply to let gravity help with the task of getting as much semen through the cervix as possible. Some people suggest that placing a pillow under the woman's hips and keeping her legs raised after sex may enhance the sperm's ability to swim upstream. You can, of course, get pregnant having intercourse in almost any position, but there are certain gravity-defying positions, such as sitting, standing, or woman on top, that may discourage sperm from traveling upstream.

Related to this issue is the ongoing debate about whether female orgasm helps in conception. The theory is that the contractions of the uterus that accompany orgasm "suck" semen up through the cervix and help propel sperm along their way into the fallopian tubes. Actual evidence for this theory, however, is lacking.[57] Of course, it's a lot more fun for the woman if she has an orgasm (or, better yet, orgasms). Anything that makes sex more likely is going to help a couple's chances for conception, so from that standpoint, you can say that female orgasm is good for fertility.

What about when you do not want to get pregnant, which for most women will be the majority of their lives? If you're not on the Pill, what type of condoms should you be on the lookout for? Are there any condoms that guys like more than others?

☞ When a guy buys some condoms, he's usually looking for something that won't feel like a condom (unless he's looking for a way to delay his ejaculation, in which case he'll have the opposite perspective). The main reasons guys don't like condoms is that they dull the sensations from their penis to some degree and, of course, they require a pause in the action in order to get one on. He also wants a condom that fits—too tight or too baggy doesn't work. Other features—such as lubrication, addition of a spermicide, colors, and flavors—are less important, generally speaking.

With all that said, there aren't any rigorous, randomized surveys of what kinds of condoms guys like. But one online marketer of condoms, undercovercondoms.com, created an online customer-feedback survey to collect this information. They created a ranking of their customers' 10 favorite condoms using a carefully weighted formula that takes into account sales volume, customer reviews, and other factors such as repeat-purchase analysis. Here's what they found:

Rank	Product name	Popularity index
1.	Trojan Magnum Lubricated	250
2.	Lifestyles Snugger Fit	237
3.	Trojan Magnum XL Lubricated	227
4.	Durex Avanti	109
5.	Trojan SUPRA Spermicidal Lubricated	78
6.	Trojan Non-Lubricated	75
7.	Trojan Shared Pleasure Warm Sensations	69
8.	Okamoto Beyond Seven	68
9.	Okamoto Crown Skin Less Skin	61
10.	Durex Extra Sensitive	61

What about the sheepskin condom? Do people actually use these things? They sound gross.

☞ They're not as gross as they sound, and yes, they're actually made from a natural pouch in the small intestine of a sheep. There's only one brand on the market right now (Trojan Naturalamb). They're not for everyone. For one thing, they're slightly "baggy" on most guys, which you either love or hate. But some guys swear they get more feeling from "skins" than from even the new types of ultrathin condoms. One big problem with these babies, however, is that they protect only against pregnancy—*not* sexually transmitted diseases such as HIV. Because they're made from animal skin, they contain small pores, which are small enough to block sperm. But sperm are like blue whales compared with virus particles, which zip merrily through the holes in a skin condom while all the "whales" are stopped dead in their tracks.

Instead of asking a guy to swathe his penis in sheepskin, how about male birth-control pills? We keep hearing about research, but then nothing ever seems to happen—what's going on? You would think guys would love to pop a pill rather than use condoms. Is there any hope?

☞ Don't hold your breath. It turns out that it's a heck of a lot easier to try to manipulate or thwart the one egg a woman normally releases each month than the hundreds of millions of sperm a guy produces every single day. Even if a method is 99 percent effective in killing or blocking sperm, that would still leave more than a million little guys in each ejaculate ready and raring to go in their effort to impregnate a woman.

That said, research into a male contraceptive is moving ahead. The most promising approach, rather ironically, involves using high doses of testosterone. That's right. As I mentioned earlier, testosterone at above-normal levels shuts down the sperm-making machinery.

Current research is looking at injections of a combination of testosterone and another sex hormone, progesterone. In parts of Europe and Canada, clinical trials are testing the effectiveness and safety of this combination. But clearly, a method involving injections isn't going to be very popular. And this type of contraception would do nothing to protect a man (or woman) from sexually transmitted diseases.

I know that women who are trying to conceive are told they should take folic acid supplements. Are there any vitamins or supplements that would help a guy be more fertile?

☞ You've hit on an area of some debate. Several years ago, studies strongly suggested that antioxidant vitamins such as C and E can reduce the amount of chromosomal damage in a guy's sperm. More recent work, however, suggests that although some chromosomal damage may be reduced, high doses of such vitamins may actually hurt sperm chromosomes in other ways.[58]

That doesn't mean vitamins aren't good for you. I always recommend that guys who want to be healthy take a daily multivitamin that gives them 100 percent of the recommended levels of required vitamins and minerals in addition to antioxidants such as vitamins A, C, and E and selenium, and zinc. These are *not* the same as megadoses of vitamins. Megadoses are most likely to be useless (your body simply excretes the excess), but in some cases they can actually be harmful. Vitamin C, for example, is ascorbic acid. Taken at high doses, the acid can really disrupt your stomach and make any predisposition to ulcers worse.

Fertility will improve as a guy's overall health improves. Men (and women) should eat a healthy diet that is very low in processed foods, sugar, and refined starches such as white flour. The latest research shows that simple carbohydrates are what's bad for you, not so much fat or natural carbs such as those found in fruits and veggies. If you make your own food, as opposed to eating fast food or highly processed frozen foods, you'll not only enjoy eating more, you'll be a lot more healthy.

We really should talk about the most common form of contraception out there—menstruation! Nothing says romance quite like cramps and bloating. Most women I know hate to have sex while on their periods, and guys don't really love ending up with bloody penises, either. What about guys—obviously, they don't bleed, but do they have PMS-y cycles similar to women's? When my husband's in a bad mood, I accuse him of being on his "male period." (He loves it!)

☞ As I discussed earlier, testosterone levels do vary daily, with levels generally highest in the mornings. But these have only a marginal effect on sex drive and even less to do with mood.

The cycles related to mood (aside from the menstrual cycle) are those of blood sugar levels, tension, and tiredness. Men and women frequently become more irritable, short-tempered, and "bitchy" when their blood sugar levels sag.[59] The problem is compounded by fatigue and complicated by tension. When energy is low and tension is high—as is typical in the late afternoon and before dinnertime—watch out! Parents of small children know this time as the "witching hour," but it applies to the parents as well as the kids.

Is there less of a chance of pregnancy if the man ejaculates just inside the vagina, as opposed to all the way inside the vagina, near the cervix?

☞ Given the ability of sperm to swim vigorously, it won't make a big difference where a guy ejaculates in the vagina, though, of course, the optimal place is right against the cervix. Since it's rather unlikely that a guy is going to keep his penis motionless in the outer part of the vagina, even if he did ejaculate there, a couple of extra thrusts will push some of the semen farther into the vagina.

Do men with larger penises have a better chance of impregnating a woman than a man with a smaller penis?

☞ No—within the normal range of penis sizes it makes absolutely no difference. Only if the penis is really tiny—under 3 inches when erect, the condition discussed earlier called microphallus—would fertility be impaired.

Assuming fertility isn't an issue, what about gender? Some couples seem to have kids of only one sex—no matter how many they have. You know, the family who keeps trying for an adorable little girl and ends up with three rowdy little boys. Do some guys just produce one gender or the other?

☞ It's dimly possible that some kind of as-yet-unknown genetic fluke predisposes some guys to produce kids of only one gender. Much more likely, however, is that "runs" of same-sex kids are just the workings of random chance. Most people have only a foggy idea of what true randomness looks like. They think that, in the case of coin tossing, a random occurrence would mean something like a head, a tail, a head, a head, a tail, and so on. In fact, in any truly random phenomenon, there are "runs" of results. Try flipping a coin a hundred times. It's highly likely that you'll get at least one run of four heads or four tails in a row. Flip the coin enough, and you'll find longer and longer runs—though, of course, they won't happen very often. In a population of hundreds of millions of couples, it would be highly unusual for there not to be families of, say, eight girls, or seven boys, or whatever. That's how randomness works, and it's the most likely explanation for such seemingly unusual families.

Can one man's sperm be more "potent" than another's? Does the "swimming" ability of each man's sperm differ? Is there any way to tell?

☞ Absolutely. The medical term is "motility." Guys whose sperm swim like junior Olympians have high motility. The guys with couch-potato sperm have low motility. The sperm made in men with small testicles tend to have lower motility and other abnormalities, in addition to having fewer sperm overall.

One common cause of low motility is a varicocele— the set of enlarged veins we discussed earlier. Men with significant varicoceles sometimes have one testicle smaller than the other. Men with varicoceles can also have "low-hanging fruit." These can be signs of a problem with a guy's fertility.

Most women have heard that the withdrawal method of birth control—where your partner pulls out just before his orgasm so the semen doesn't land inside of you—is pretty much a joke. Why?

☞ It's because a guy doesn't have to ejaculate to get you pregnant. Most men "leak" a substance commonly referred to as "precome." This pre-ejaculate is made up of somewhat sticky, clear fluid from the prostate. Sperm are present in this fluid and, therefore, you could get pregnant even if the guy swears up and down that he didn't ejaculate. So no matter what, if there is an unprotected penis inside your vagina, there is always a possibility of becoming pregnant.

What if you do want to get pregnant? Let's say I've bought What to Expect When You're Expecting, *I'm tracking my cycle like a broker tracks his stocks, and I'm popping folic acid along with the multivit-amins. I'd like my husband to pull his weight, too.*

☞ There are plenty of things he should do—or not do—to be as fertile as possible:

➡ What is bad for the heart is bad for the testicles and penis, and for fertility. Your partner should maintain a proper weight and exercise. Overweight men have a 20 percent greater chance of being infertile, as well as an increased chance of heart disease and diabetes. He should also stop smoking. Smoking hurts the blood vessels of the heart and those of the penis and testicles.

➡ Lower cholesterol levels are associated with better erectile function. Make sure your partner's cholesterol is under control, either by eating sensibly or taking a cholesterol-lowering medication.

➡ Smaller waist size (with increased muscle weight) increases testosterone—resulting in better fertility and better sex.

➡ Don't let your partner take hot baths or get into Jacuzzis—it's the equivalent of dunking testicles in hot water like a tea bag.

➡ Make sure he's eating a well-balanced diet. If he's overweight, limit bread, pizza, pasta, cookies, and cake. Also limit added sugar and salt, and add a daily multivitamin and the basic antioxidants.

➡ He should exercise 5 days a week for 45 minutes a day. Specifically, I recommend aerobic activity such as a treadmill or elliptical machine at two-thirds maximum heart rate for 45 minutes, 5 days a week. Resistance training (such as weight lifting) 2 days a week will help, too. Exercising the lower body, from the waist down, will increase the muscle mass and increase the blood flow to the pelvis and groin (testicles and penis). This will markedly decrease the chance of erectile dysfunction.

➡ Avoid lubricants when having sex, since lubricants decrease sperm movement and can result in infertility.

➡ Guys should avoid anabolic steroids at all costs. They radically decrease sperm counts and soften and sometimes shrink the testicles.

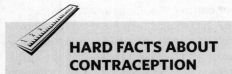

HARD FACTS ABOUT CONTRACEPTION

Speed at which sperm swim: about 4 millimeters per second, or roughly 47 feet per hour

Speed at which Olympic swimmer Michael Phelps swims: roughly 20,000 feet per hour (4 mph) doing his fastest stroke

Number of sperm that come out during the typical ejaculation: 200 million

Best sexual position for getting pregnant: missionary

TROUBLESHOOTING

Erectile Dysfunction and Other Bedroom Problems

IN THE THORNY LAND of libido, nothing is a bigger buzz-kill than premature ejaculation or its demon cousin, the lost erection. It's easy for us, as women, to think it's something we did. If my boyfriend were really attracted to me, you might think, he wouldn't go limp whenever we're about to do it. It makes you feel ugly. It's somewhat insulting. And, let's face it, you also wind up feeling extremely sexually frustrated. I've seen several relationships implode because the guy simply couldn't maintain an erection. You can try to work your way around it with substitutes, like oral sex, cuddling, or long talks—but at the end of the day, you're postponing the inevitable. When a guy can't nail you, it's usually the last nail in the coffin of your relationship.

Premature ejaculation isn't much better. It's awkward and humiliating for the guy, who feels like an overexcited twelve-year-old staring at a pair of breasts for the first time, and we're left pulling out the box of tissues—if not to dry his eyes, then to dry our sheets. It also makes us automatic liars. "It happens to all guys," we say. Or perhaps this: "Really, it's not a big deal. I just like being close to you." And sure, every now and then, it's okay. Maybe he's had too much to drink and can't get it up. Maybe he hasn't gotten laid in a while and is simply just bursting with semen. But if you always feel like you're going to bed with an overactive volcano or a 90-year-old man, you need help.

Fortunately, it's not the end of the world. Before you launch into a deep psychological probe of your relationship or begin to wonder why you're the most repulsive creature God ever created, brush up on some biology.

So, Harry, we all think we know premature ejaculation when we see it (or feel it), but what does premature really mean?

☞ Premature ejaculation (PE) is the number one male sexual problem. But when, exactly, is an ejaculation "premature"? It's difficult to pin down, because it all depends on what the partners involved desire and expect. What's "premature" for one couple might be just right for another. The formal definition, therefore, avoids specifying a time limit: Premature ejaculation is simply ejaculation that regularly occurs sooner than desired, either before or shortly after penetration, causing distress to one or both partners.

How many guys out there actually have this problem?

☞ Defined this way, about one in three men between the ages of 18 and 60 experience premature ejaculation. Some men are so sensitive they ejaculate before their penis has even entered a woman's vagina. Others climax within seconds of entry. A review published in 2007 found that 87 percent of men with premature ejaculation reported that they climaxed within 2 minutes of vaginal entry. (That compares with only 22 percent of guys without PE.) The studies of what is a "normal" length of time for a guy to have vaginal intercourse before ejaculating produce rather wide-ranging results. Kinsey reported that about 75 percent of guys ejaculate within 2 minutes, which he noted is "a frequent source of marital conflict." More recent studies find longer times. One study of U.S. men found an average of 9.2 minutes. Another study conducted in five European countries found an average of 5.4 minutes.[60] (And if you're wondering how these times are obtained, it's via the use of a stopwatch by the study participants.)

I can understand younger guys having ejaculation issues. I mean, they're delicate, innocent flowers—and seeing a woman naked is still a novelty. They can't contain their excitement. Fine. But what happens when guys get more mature?

☞ Premature ejaculation does tend to resolve with age— the male biological clock slows down the sexual response cycle. But this usually happens long after a great deal of sexual dissatisfaction has occurred for the unfortunate man and his partners. Fortunately, premature ejaculation is one of the easiest problems to treat today. The most common approach is to use very low doses of antidepressants that are known to delay orgasm. Effective doses range from about half the normal daily dose to doses typically used in depressed patients. The orgasm-delaying effects of these drugs occur within about four hours, which means men can use them periodically if they want. Some men, however, prefer to simply take a pill a day so they don't have to think about it and can respond more spontaneously to romantic situations.

But what if your husband/boyfriend/lover/friend-with-benefits doesn't want to take an antidepressant? That seems excessive and a bit drama queen–ish, don't you think? Suggesting a Zoloft prescription to a guy is right up there with saying "We need to talk" or "I want you to meet my grandmother" as a surefire man-alienator. Although, if a guy is having these kinds of issues, maybe he could use some cheering up.

☞ Well, there are other approaches. One is to use one of a variety of anesthetic creams that mildly numb the penis and so delay orgasm. The creams must be used carefully, since too much of them can cause erections to fail from lack of feeling. If used without a condom, a cream may also cause vaginal numbness in the partner. Condoms alone can reduce penile sensation sufficiently in some men with premature ejaculation to result in satisfactory sex. In this case, you're killing many birds with one stone: preventing pregnancy, preventing some STIs, *and* prolonging intercourse!

Okay, what about erections that go missing mid-sex? This is even worse than premature ejaculation, I think. I mean, at least with a premature ejaculation, you know the guy is interested in you. Maybe too interested in you. But it's so easy to think that a guy who loses his erection inside of you just caught a glimpse of your back fat or something. There's nothing like a boner gone bad to make a woman feel undesirable.

☞ The penis has a mind of its own. Leonardo da Vinci once sagely observed of the male organ: "Many times the man wishes it to practice and it does not wish it; many times it wishes it and the man forbids it." The simple fact is that all men, at one time or another, will lose their erection just when they want it most. The factors that contribute to this include fatigue, stress, tension, illness, distraction, and boredom. Or they had one drink too many, or had too much coffee, or they're taking a prescription medication that impairs erections (and there are many of those). The list of specific drugs is so long, we don't have room for it here. Instead, here's a list of broad classes of medications known to contribute to erectile or orgasm problems:

➡ SSRI antidepressants
➡ Blood pressure medications
➡ Sedatives
➡ Antianxiety drugs
➡ Narcotics
➡ Stimulants
➡ Estrogens
➡ Some ulcer medications

Of course, sometimes the benefits of a drug outweigh any adverse effects on sex. If a guy thinks that a medica-

...ion may be causing a problem, he should talk to his doctor about it. Sometimes other medications with different
side-effect profiles can be tried.

Unfortunately, an instance or two of erectile failure
can mutate into a more stubborn problem. An instance
of erectile dysfunction usually begins as a purely physical problem with blood vessels, nerves, or other parts of
the male reproductive machinery. But very rapidly a
complicated psychological dimension is layered onto
the physical problem—which almost always makes
things worse.

*You mean, you end up with a guy who needs constant coaxing and
reassurance that he can perform. A few unsuccessful sex sessions
and you turn into a motivational speaker, living in a van, down by
the river . . .*

☞ Yup. Performance anxiety sets in. And, since anxiety
releases hormones that clamp down blood vessels, fear
of failure becomes a self-fulfilling prophecy. The resulting sexual snowball can lead to less and less sex, feelings of emotional distance, abandonment, rejection,
and anger.

Sex therapy can be helpful for this problem. Sometimes just being able to talk about it with one's partner
relieves some of the anxiety at the root of the problem.
Couples can also learn ways to be more relaxed about
sex, which, again, can alleviate the tension. And, of
course, there are various erection-enhancing drugs available that can allow a man to feel more confident that his
erection will be reliable. The only hazard of using drugs
like Viagra in this case is that a guy could become psy-
chologically dependent on them.

How should women react, ideally, when a guy has trouble getting up or ejaculates too soon? So often guys feel berated and put down by their partners when this happens. (And women don't feel amazing, either.) Harry, what are your tips for proper bedroom dialogue when things go wrong?

☞ There are a couple of things that can help. First of all, it really helps to have a sense of humor. This is sex, after all, not brain surgery. If you can lighten up about an instance where things don't go smoothly, you'll both be much more likely to be able to talk about it. And talking is really key. Maybe there's something about the way you both approach sex that could be changed so that the guy will either not lose his erection or won't come so fast. For example, some guys will lose their erection while giving a woman oral stimulation. As lovely as cunnilingus can be, it can also take some time, and while his mouth is fully occupied with giving you pleasure, his penis may simply take a nap. That's just an example— there could be all sorts of other little "turnoffs" going on for one or both of you that you won't discover unless you talk freely about it.

What's most helpful isn't something specific that you say, but the way you say it. Showing that it's not a huge deal and that you care about the guy regardless of whether you have sex this time can relieve a great deal of stress and allow the guy to relax. Assure the guy that this isn't about performance or perfection. Things just go wrong sometimes, and the best approach (at least at first) is to accept it and not get too frustrated.

Of course, if a problem becomes chronic and nothing you try seems to make any difference, then you can consider other options, such as having the guy use an erection-enhancing medication, going to sex therapy, or finding someone with whom you're more sexually compatible.

Let's assume that a woman is dating a guy who always loses his erection under certain circumstances—say, for instance, every time he gets drunk. (Why she's dating a guy who drinks to this point is a different story.) How is it that alcohol makes guys horny but not hard?

☞ The porter in *Macbeth* gets it right when he says that drink "provokes the desire, but takes away the performance." Research shows that by most physical measures alcohol is bad for sex. Scientists have measured how alcohol affects penile swelling, vaginal engorgement, time required to achieve orgasm (both during intercourse and masturbation), and vaginal lubrication. The results are strikingly uniform: Alcohol inhibited all of these sexual responses. Erections are slower to rise and quicker to fall, vaginas are slower to lubricate, and orgasms are slower to arrive.

But nothing is simple when it comes to alcohol. "Whiskey penis" (and "whiskey clitoris") occurs at relatively high blood alcohol levels—equivalent to what you might expect after three or four drinks consumed in a short period of time. When the alcohol levels are lower, things change. A drink or two to "loosen up" may, indeed, help sexual performance. In part, that's because an erection requires the relaxing of the arteries feeding the penis, and a modest dose of alcohol can help this along. In addition, some people expect alcohol to help them respond sexually, and this belief can be as powerful as the alcohol itself.

This phenomenon was demonstrated in one of the classic experiments in the field.[61] The sexual arousal of four groups of male college students was measured while they watched an erotic video. Students in one group drank a vodka and tonic before watching and were told the truth about the drink. Another group got disguised tonic but were told it contained vodka. The third group actually got alcohol but were told it was just tonic water. And the last group got just tonic water and were told the truth about it.

The results? The most aroused group was the guys who drank alcohol and knew it. But the guys who believed they got alcohol when they didn't were significantly more aroused than those who thought they were drinking only tonic water but actually consumed vodka. The belief was more potent than the alcohol, in other words—though, clearly, alcohol did contribute to the arousal in guys who had it.

So let's say you're having a tequila-fueled sex session and, suddenly, the guy's penis goes limp. Will coffee help?

☞ Nope—it'll actually make things worse. Although if caffeine made it really hard to get hard, it wouldn't be the world's favorite drug (which it is). One way that caffeine works is by plugging up a molecule that tends to slow things down. It's a lot like putting a brick under your brake pedal: You end up going faster because you can't slow down. That's great when you want to speed up your brain, but caffeine travels throughout your body.

And, among other things, it interferes with the ability of blood vessels to relax and open up. When this happens in hands or feet, they get cooler than normal because less blood is flowing—but at least you can still use them. It's another story with the penis.

For a penis striving for erection, blood supply is everything. The normal state of affairs for a penis is that the arteries feeding it are clamped down by surrounding muscles. This keeps the penis soft, small (or smaller), and out of harm's way. If the arteries open up—bingo—the penis fills like the sponge that it is, and it's ready for action. So you can see the problem with caffeine. All those caffeine molecules are like tiny clamps on the penile arteries, choking off the blood needed to get a man hard. And if he does manage to get it up, the caffeine is still there, making it much more likely that he'll wilt at the slightest interruption, distraction, or loss of direct stimulation.

Now, having said all that, we're still talking about a general influence here. A teenage boy is unlikely to see any difference in his erectile function even after chugging five Red Bulls in a row. Caffeine's impact on a guy's erection becomes more acute as he gets older.

How about marijuana? After all, sometimes that's the preferred drug, not booze.

☞ As most people who have tried marijuana know, one of its effects is to increase the intensity of sensory stimuli. That means that the sense of touch and sexuality can be as heightened as one's appreciation of music or visual stimuli. Very simply put, marijuana is thought to enhance sex and that's one of the reasons it's such a popular drug.

The degree to which marijuana use can impair health is directly related to the amount used. In very general terms, marijuana is not as toxic or as potentially addictive as alcohol and other recreational drugs. Among the conclusions of the landmark study by the Institute of Medicine:

Marijuana is not a completely benign substance. It is a powerful drug with a variety of effects. However, except for the harm associated with smoking, the adverse effects of marijuana use are within the range tolerated for other medications.[62]

Nonetheless, couples interested in conceiving a baby would be wise to avoid marijuana because it does exert some potentially harmful effects on fertility—effects that increase with the dosage consumed. For example, studies in both animals and humans show that marijuana use is associated with declines in luteinizing hormone, which controls the production of both testosterone and estrogen.[63] THC, the major active agent in marijuana, has also been shown to interfere with the implantation of embryos in the uterine wall. For these and other reasons, therefore, it's best to avoid marijuana (and avoid smoking tobacco and drinking alcohol, too, of course) if you want to preserve your fertility.

What about peeing problems? If a guy is having a tough time going to the bathroom, is he also going to have a tough time ejaculating?

☞ If a guy's having a hard time peeing, he ought to get checked out, because something's wrong. He might have a urinary tract infection, which might affect his ejaculation, depending on where the infection is. Alternatively, his prostate might be enlarged. This is fairly common in men as they age. It's called benign prostatic hyperplasia, or BPH. It's not the same thing as cancer, and often the swelling doesn't produce any signs at all. But it can constrict the urethra, making it harder to pee, among other things. To date, however, there's been no evidence that BPH interferes with either erections or ejaculation.[64]

This talk of prostates has got me thinking. . . . Let's discuss older guys for a minute. What do we have to look forward to? Does erectile dysfunction increase as you get older?

☞ Yes. There's a very clear, steady rise in the incidence of ED with age. Only about 10 percent of men in their thirties report ED, but the percentage goes up about 10 percent a decade after that. In one study, 70 percent of guys in their early seventies reported some degree of ED.[65] High blood pressure, high cholesterol levels, and diabetes all raise a guy's risk of ED, regardless of his age.

Which is where drugs like Viagra come in, right? Even if your bedmate isn't a cholesterol-ridden diabetic, can ED drugs enhance the sexual experience?

☞ Many people think that Viagra and other medications for ED make men, to put it scientifically, horny. Not exactly. They all block an enzyme in the penis, which ends up relaxing the blood vessels. More blood = faster boners. Horniness, or libido, on the other hand, has nothing to do with plumbing and everything to do with testosterone. Since none of the erection-enhancing drugs has any effect on testosterone, they don't directly increase libido. Of course, if a guy is made much more confident in his erectile prowess because of a pill, then he might appear more horny.

Having said that, there is one important connection between Viagra and other erection-boosters and testosterone. For reasons that are still unclear, guys with unusually low testosterone levels don't respond as well to the ED medications. Any man who thinks he needs a medication to help him perform should see a doctor instead of browsing the Internet for good deals. Erectile dysfunction can be an important telltale sign of other diseases, such as diabetes and high blood pressure. Viagra, in other words, shouldn't be a quick fix for a larger issue. As for the sex: It's not as if Viagra changes the way the penis feels to the guy. It's the same penis, just hard. The feelings of orgasm and ejaculation are the same, too. But the overall experience of sex can be quite different—and much better—because a guy can remain more reliably hard and may be able to obtain another erection after the ejaculatory latency period much faster. As many men tell me, that kind of sex "feels like the old days."

Can women take ED drugs to feel more intense orgasms?

☞ Yes, women can take drugs meant to enhance male erections, but they may, or may not, feel more-intense orgasms. Basically, a penis is, anatomically speaking, just a giant clitoris. All of the basic parts are the same—shaft and head, for example—and the relatively tiny clitoris contains just as many sensory nerve endings as the much larger penis. The clitoris, too, becomes erect during sexual excitation, and since this is a matter of blood vessels, the drugs that relax those vessels in a man do the same thing in women.

Some studies of Viagra in women have found a benefit in terms of a woman's ability to become aroused, achieve orgasm, and enjoy sex.[66] But other studies did not find a benefit, so the jury is still out.

Will ED drugs improve a guy's fertility?

☞ Not directly. ED drugs have no effect on sperm counts or quality. Only in those rare cases where a couple is "infertile" because a man can't achieve an erection might ED drugs be of some help.

Do some guys just have naturally limper penises than others?

☞ There may be some variation in the "tone" of erect penises, but it is not significant. More common is that the rigidity and "height" of a man's erection slowly decline with age.

This may sound like a silly question, but if the penis fills with blood during an erection, how come the penis doesn't actually bleed during ejaculation?

☞ The blood that fills a penis during erection is contained within three cylindrical, fingerlike regions of spongy tis-

sue, which is physically contained within a tough
very flexible) covering. Semen (and urine) are carr,
though a tube called the urethra, which is also physical
separate from the "guts" of a penis. Hence there is no
chance for any penile blood to enter the urethra in a
normal, undamaged penis.

*Do men go to the urologist like women go to the gynecologist, get-
ting checkups every year? Or do they just go when they're having
problems?*

☞ Actually, guys don't go to the doctor even when
they're having problems. I can't count the number of
times a guy has come to my office and said his wife or
partner insisted he see me. Guys tend to simply avoid
encounters that are likely to involve their genitals.
That's a real problem, of course, because many problems are much more easily solved if they are caught
early.

Ideally, guys would see their doctor every year for a
general physical. This typically includes a digital rectal
examination of the prostate—the doctor inserts a
gloved, lubricated finger into the anus and feels the size
and texture of the prostate. It's not exactly something
most guys look forward to, but it's fast and painless and
far simpler than pelvic exams. Another part of an exam
is a general inspection of the male genitals and a check
of the testicles for any irregularities.

All in all, guys have it pretty easy when it comes to
physical exams, and I always tell them they shouldn't
complain about it—and certainly not to their wife or female partner!

ASK A GUY

Can sexual incompatibility ruin an erection?

Yes. I was with an overly aggressive woman who kept trying to bite me in bed. It was our first time together. We were a little drunk. And even though I kept pushing her away, she kept trying to bite me hard. I lost my hard-on almost instantly and had difficulty getting it back. Nothing helps an erection more than being turned on by the woman you're with. Nothing kills an erection more than the woman doing something that you find inappropriate or even gross.

THE ITCHY AND SCRATCHY SHOW

Sexually Transmitted Infections (STIs)

I'M LUCKY. I SUCCESSFULLY navigated my dating years without coming into contact with a single STI. But that doesn't mean I haven't worried about 'em. Actually, worried is too mild a word. Several years ago, I had a self-induced nervous breakdown in which I convinced myself that I had HIV. This episode climaxed (for lack of a better term) with the man who is now my husband getting his penis prodded with a Q-tip and me threatening bodily harm to a kindly nurse at my local doctor's office. Let me explain.

It all started innocently enough. When I first began dating my husband, I was so excited to sleep with someone I actually liked that I wasn't as careful as perhaps I should have been. He looked clean. He said he was clean. Blinded by passion (and maybe a few too many rum and Cokes), my better judgment went over the side of the bed along with my brand-new Victoria's Secret bra, and we had unprotected sex. I was on the Pill, after all. So, really, I had nothing to worry about. Things like herpes, genital warts, chlamydia, HIV—those things happened to unfortunate people in health-ed textbooks. Not to me.

My innocence was shattered at a party one evening when my husband's particularly gossipy neighbor cornered me next to the keg. She pulled me aside and said, "You know that Brian slept with Laurie, right?" Well, yes, thank goodness, I already knew that.

"Of course," I replied.

"Well, I just want you to know—and I'm telling you this as a friend—that basically everyone has slept with her." She smiled meanly at me. "You should probably get tested."

At that point, I had to exercise serious self-control not to vomit in my little red plastic beer cup. Brian had told me about his dalliance with Laurie, but he didn't tell me she had been ridden more times than Space Mountain. I immediately became convinced that every STI known to man (or woman) was coursing through my bloodstream. I sent Brian on a battery of tests. Defeated, he reported to me that a rude male nurse had violated him with a Q-tip. I didn't feel an ounce of sympathy. I marched myself to the gynecologist and spread my legs in desperation. She tried to reassure me that I probably didn't have HIV—or any other STI, for that matter. She swabbed me, blood-tested me, then she said she'd be in touch in two weeks.

Two weeks?! They were the longest two weeks of my life. I spent my days envisioning genital warts where they didn't exist. I spent my nights surfing the Internet for symptoms. Finally, a message from my doctor's office: "Hi, this is Nurse Ruthanne calling. We have your blood test results back. Please call the doctor at your earliest conv—"

I slammed the phone down. *Holy crap! I must be dying.* If I was okay, she would have just said I was fine, right? I dialed the number and expected the Grim Reaper to answer. "Hello, you careless whore. We have a special brothel in hell for girls like you!" Instead, I got good ol' Ruthanne on the first ring. "I'm sorry," she told me. *Sorry?* "The doctor is with a patient now. I can't release your information. The doctor must speak to you directly." I began to cry. I begged, cajoled, wept, and, yes, threatened. I'm not sure, but I think I called Ruthanne a cocktease. Finally, she caved. Her voice dropped to a whisper. "Honey, I'm not supposed to do this," she clucked. "But—well—all I can say is don't worry. Get my meaning? You don't have to worry." I wasn't going to die! Hooray! I did a little dance alone in my bedroom.

Today, I'm many years older and many years wiser. And I'd like to help you avoid enduring your own version of my self-created melodrama. Read on.

First things first: How reliable are STI tests? All this time, I thought I was clean—for the sake of my marriage, please don't turn me back into a paranoid wreck!

☞ Breathe easy. While no medical test is 100 percent accurate, clinic-based tests for STIs are certainly accurate enough to rely upon. There are many different tests for each of the different STIs. Some STIs are hard to test for if you don't have any symptoms. Some STIs can be tested through blood work, urine tests, or saliva tests.

Other STIs can only be tested by culturing a sample of body fluid from the penis, vagina, rectum, or open sore.

Home testing kits are available for HIV, herpes, chlamydia, and gonorrhea. Most involve mailing a sample or swab to a laboratory for testing. But beware of fraudulent testing kits. Several types of unapproved home-test kits have been flagged by the FDA over the years, and more are undoubtedly available via the Internet. Ask your doctor to recommend a home test if that is what you're interested in.

ASK A GUY

Can something else be mistaken for genital warts?

A girlfriend of mine once accused me of having genital warts. I was shocked. I went to the doctor to get an exam and was found to have a skin tag—those mole-like tags of flesh—on my genitalia. She thought this tag was a wart. Not surprisingly, the relationship didn't last very long.

Many women think that giving men oral sex is actually safer than vaginal sex. Can women still get infections from mouth-to-penis contact?

☞ The real question should be, What kind of infection can't you get from oral sex? The fact is, a woman can get practically any sexually transmitted infection from fellatio. Here's the list of the most common things you don't want to get:

➡ Human papillomaviruses (viruses live on the skin of the penis)

➡ Gonorrhea (bacteria are carried in semen)

➡ AIDS/HIV (virus is carried in semen)

➡ Hepatitis B (virus is carried in blood and could be passed through a small scrape, cut, or sore on the penis)

➡ Genital herpes (virus lives on skin of penis and elsewhere and can be transmitted even if a sore is not visible)

➡ Syphilis (bacteria can be transmitted from an active sore on the penis)

Gah! All the usual suspects—so much for that theory. So we'll ask this question: Are there any infections that are less likely with oral sex?

☞ The one relatively common STI that a woman is unlikely to get by performing fellatio is trichomoniasis, an infection with a single-celled parasite called a trichomonad. This little beastie resides in and around the vulva, and for transmission to occur you need either vulva-to-vulva contact or penis-to-vulva contact. In other words, a guy can carry the parasite inside his urethra and infect a woman by having intercourse with her, but you're unlikely to get the parasite by licking/sucking a guy's penis or by swallowing his semen.[67]

Speaking of parasites, let's talk about crabs. I have to admit, when I think about sexually transmitted crabs, I picture the friendly little hermit crabs we used to keep in my fourth-grade classroom dodging in and out of pubic hair. What are crabs? Are they really itty-bitty . . . crabs?

☞ They actually do sort of look like crabs under a micro-scope, but they're totally unrelated to the sea creatures. "Crabs" are really insects called pubic lice. They're re-lated to other species of lice. These insects simply have a preference for pubic hair and tend to be passed on by pubic-to-pubic contact. They can also be acquired through contact with an infected person's bed linens, towels, or clothes, as the lice can survive for up to two days without a human host.

The adult lice lay eggs, or "nits," on hair shafts near the skin. The eggs, which are white or yellow and oval shaped, hatch in approximately 7 to 10 days. The baby lice then feed on human blood. This causes the intense itching, particularly at night, that is the classic sign of pubic lice.

Ah, now I know why Brazilian waxes are so popular. If you do get crabs, what happens? Can you take a nice hot shower and scrub them off?

☞ Pubic lice and nits are not killed by ordinary soap and water, so an insecticide is needed—usually a 1 percent solution of Permethrin, which is available without a pre-scription. A single treatment is usually enough to stop an infestation.

That's reassuring. But crabs sort of seem like something people got in the 1940s after too much "heavy petting." They're definitely one of the lower-profile STIs. I think we all want to know about the more common ones.

☞ First a little background. Sexually transmitted infec-tions are extremely common. More than half of Ameri-cans will have an STI at some point in their lifetime.[68]

Every year about 9 million people contract an STI, almost half of them young people aged 15 to 24. As for prevalence, take a look at the table below, which has figures from 2000 for men and women between the ages of 15 and 24:[69]

Sexually transmitted infection	New cases in 2000
Human papillomavirus (HPV)	4.6 million
Trichomoniasis	1.9 million
Chlamydia	1.5 million
Genital herpes	640,000
Gonorrhea	431,000
HIV	15,000
Syphilis	8,200
Hepatitis B	7,500
Total	9.1 million

The dreaded, ubiquitous HPV! It seems like everyone has it or knows someone who does. How easy is it to get HPV?

☞ It's incredibly easy to get HPV, for two simple reasons: Millions of folks are infected and most infected people don't know that they are. Human papillomavirus is actually a single name for a whole group of related viruses that can infect the genitals and anus of a man or woman and the linings of the vagina and cervix. Most people who become infected with HPV will not have any symptoms and will clear the infection on their own.

But some HPV viruses are considered "high-risk" types and may cause abnormal Pap tests. They may also lead to cancer of the cervix, vulva, vagina, anus, or penis. Others are called "low-risk" types, and they may cause mild Pap test abnormalities or genital warts. Genital warts are single or multiple growths or bumps that appear in the genital area; some are cauliflower-shaped. (Yes, they are pretty gross, but not deadly.)

There is no cure for HPV infection, although in most women the infection goes away on its own. The treatments provided are directed to the changes in the skin or mucous membranes caused by HPV infection, such as warts and precancerous changes in the cervix.

Wait a sec. I've seen the commercials. I thought there was a cure— or at least a vaccine.

☞ Four of the most common HP viruses can now be prevented by a vaccine: types 16 and 18 (two "high-risk" HPVs that cause 70 percent of cervical cancers) and types 6 and 11, which cause 90 percent of genital warts.

The vaccine is recommended for girls ages 12 and 13 and any girls who have not become sexually active. Older women may benefit, too, because few women have been exposed to all four of the viruses thwarted by the vaccine. Sounds like boring advice, but the best course of action if you're interested in any of this is to visit your doctor. And remember, this vaccine does nothing for all the other types of infections you could get from sex, so you shouldn't change what you do to protect yourself.

As with so much when it comes to sex, it seems like guys have it a bit easier than women—they're silent carriers of HPV, right?

☞ Not all guys are "silent carriers." About 1 percent of guys with HPV will develop genital warts, which are visible and require treatment. But it's true—the fact is that the vast majority of guys won't have any symptoms. And since there is as yet no test for infection in men (as opposed to the Pap test for women), all of these millions of guys will be unwitting carriers of the disease. They're not really luckier.

What if the guy has warts on his balls? This must mean something, right?

☞ Maybe so. If it looks like a wart and feels like a wart, it's probably a wart—in this case, a genital wart caused by one of the human papillomaviruses. The warts themselves are not infectious—though it's unlikely you'd be interested in touching them anyway. Women can get exactly the same type of warts, by the way.

    Sometimes the warts disappear on their own; other

times they get progressively worse. Warts can be removed by surgery, chemicals, or freezing. Topical creams are also available. Even after the outbreak of warts is gone, however, the person may still be infected with the virus and thus may still infect others.

What do the warts tend to look like? Describe.

☞ They are rough lumps with a cauliflower-like appearance. Genital warts often occur in clusters and can be very tiny or can spread into large masses on the penis or genital area.

HPV is scary, but I think most women are especially afraid of HIV. I've heard lots of arguments for circumcision. (My personal favorite: "If you don't get circumcised, your penis will look like an anteater.") Are circumcised guys less likely to contract HIV?

☞ Yes indeed! The reason is simple. The foreskin is delicate and can easily suffer small cuts. An uncircumcised man who has sex with someone with HIV is more likely to contract the virus because of the exposure to his blood that can occur during the "trauma" of sex. Because of possible cuts on the skin, the virus can penetrate the body more easily. Of course, a circumcised penis can also sustain cuts, which increase the possibility of HIV transmission.

Herpes is right up there with HIV as a dreaded disease. If a guy has a sore on his lip, does this mean he's got it?

☞ It's probable with a certain type of sore, but you don't want to jump to conclusions, because there are lots of other things that can cause lesions around the lips—canker sores and pimples among them.

That said, there are two main types of herpes viruses that are very common. Type 1 herpes typically causes the classic sores, called fever blisters or cold sores, around the mouth and lips—and it's by touching these sores with your own mouth or lips that the virus is passed. Type 2 herpes typically causes genital herpes and the lesions occur, obviously, on and around the genitals. But because the prevalence of oral sex is increasing, the two types are

WHEN I'M WITH YOU, EVERY DAY IS MY BIRTHDAY . . .

. . . because you give me the gift that just keeps on giving. I just have to jump in for a moment and say, what is up with those herpes medication commercials? You know the ones. There's a strapping young guy and a perky, gorgeous woman, zipped up in fleece vests, biking down a tree-lined path, and pausing at a dewy meadow to nuzzle in the grass. They don't even have pimples; how can they have herpes? And how did they find each other? Are there special dating sites for people who have herpes? Do people with herpes tend to exclusively date other people with herpes? Is it something you can try to overlook, like halitosis or a receding hairline? How do you tell someone, "Hi, I'd like to get to know you better, but if and when we consummate our relationship, I might end up giving you recurrent, unsightly sores. But I think we really connect. Your place or mine?"

increasingly crossing their typical boundaries—hence, Type 1 can cause genital herpes and Type 2 can cause the classic oral symptoms.

Once you get herpes (of either type), the virus cannot be eradicated. It lives adjacent to nerve cells, and outbreaks can occur periodically and unpredictably. Some medications are now available that can shorten an outbreak and reduce symptoms. The disease is generally treated with an antiviral drug such as acyclovir (Zovirax), or a medication such as famciclovir (Famvir) or valacyclovir (Valtrex). The antiviral drugs are most effective if the treatment begins within 72 hours of appearance of definitive symptoms.

That's why I always thought that peeing after sex was a good idea—you know, to cleanse the system and wash away sperm and other unsavories. Does it work?

☞ No! The only advantage of peeing after sex is to flush out bacteria that can cause a urinary tract infection. So it's certainly a good idea, but peeing after sex will do nothing to reduce your risk of a sexually transmitted infection, and it certainly will not prevent pregnancy.

I know UTIs don't qualify as STIs, but I know people who tend to get them when they're having a lot of sex. Should a woman be worried about a new partner's health if she gets a UTI after they start having sex? Is it a sign that he could pass something more serious along to her?

☞ Half of all women will develop a urinary tract infection (UTI) during their lifetimes, and many will experience more than one. A UTI is caused by bacteria that have entered the urinary system, usually through the urethra—which is rather unfortunately located quite near the anus, a rich source of bacteria.

Bacteria typically infect the bladder, which can be painful and annoying. Serious consequences can occur if the infection spreads to your kidneys.

For many women, especially women who go from having little sex to having lots, sexual intercourse seems to trigger an infection. Historically, this was called "honeymoon cystitis," as many women having sex for the first time during their honeymoon would get a UTI. Another potential source of an infection, however, is a man with a urinary tract infection. This isn't as uncommon as you might think, though figures are difficult to come by because many male UTIs don't provoke obvious symptoms. Contracting a UTI after sex with a new partner isn't anything to panic about, although it never hurts to get checked out if you're worried.

Usually, UTI symptoms clear up within a few days of treatment with an antibiotic. But you may need to continue antibiotics for a week or more. Take the entire course of antibiotics recommended by your doctor to ensure that the infection is completely eradicated. And if your partner is infected, he will need to take a course of antibiotics, too—otherwise, you will be passing the bacteria back and forth during sex!

So let's go back to STIs. Can you get an STI even if your partner is wearing a condom?

☞ Yes. STIs associated with semen are preventable with a condom. But about 1 percent of condoms either break or fall off. And even if the condom is perfect, it only covers the skin of the penis. If a man has skin lesions such as warts over his pubic area or thighs, that skin will still touch you, so his STI can be transmitted even when condoms are worn.

What happens if you don't treat an STI right away?

☞ As with any medical condition, the sooner you treat an STI, the easier it is to control or eradicate it and the less severe the symptoms will be. Left untreated, some STIs (such as syphilis) can be debilitating or fatal. So get treatment immediately!

Can a history of STIs render a man infertile?

☞ Possibly. Many STIs and urinary tract infections can create scarring that may, for example, block the ejaculatory ducts or the fine tubes of the epididymis. Sometimes a guy will know there's a problem because he'll feel pain during ejaculation or see some other sign of trouble. But just as often, there will be no outward sign that anything is wrong. Only when a couple can't conceive and the guy comes in for a thorough examination and evaluation will the problem be discovered.

Are some men immune to STIs? A guy I went to college with was always bragging about the amount of unprotected sex he had—and he never suffered from so much as a painful pee.

☞ Nobody's completely immune to infectious diseases, but it's certainly true that people vary in their vulnerability and the strength of their immune systems. If a guy is disease-free even though he has engaged in a lot of risky sex, then he's just plain lucky, he has a very robust immune system, or both. But sooner or later, such a guy is going to become infected.

Where do STIs originate? They had to start somewhere—perhaps with Itchius Lumpidius, the ancient god of venereal diseases?

☞ Viruses and bacteria existed on the planet long before humans and other mammals. They develop very quickly because of their very short life cycles and have thus been spread from species to species over the eons, evolving better and better ways to infect hosts, which, in turn, evolve better and better immune systems. Some definitely are serious diseases, but STI is the commonly used term now.

So why do we now say STIs, not STDs?

☞ The word "disease" was deemed to have an overly negative connotation and implied a degree of seriousness that didn't reflect some of the less deadly infections, such as chlamydia.

HARD FACTS ABOUT STIs

Man who holds the record for having sex with the most women: The late basketball player Wilt Chamberlain claimed to have slept with roughly 20,000 women. For this to be true, he would have had to have sex with more than nine women a week, starting when he was 15 and continuing for 40 years.

Percentage of women who are infertile because of untreated STIs: At least 15 percent of all infertile American women are so because of tubal damage caused by pelvic inflammatory disease (PID), the result of an untreated STI.

Most common STI: HPV

KEEPIN' IT CLEAN

Men and Hygiene

WE SAVED THE BEST for last, ladies: cleanliness. Don't you wish guys were as well-versed as women in the art of personal hygiene? For us, puberty came complete with a set of accessories: tweezers, razors, deodorant, various fruit- and flower-scented liquids. I still remember the first time I shaved my legs, using a gnarly old Bic razor that I found at the bottom of my mother's makeup bag. I felt as if I was doing something clandestine, naughty, and oh so grown up. It was a rite of passage. Clearly, if I was shaving my legs, someone might actually be looking at them. The prospect thrilled me to the core. I had acne, braces, and pegged paisley pants (the Gap was big into paisley that year, what can I say?)—but my legs were smooth, dammit.

Sadly, these glorious grooming moments are lost on most guys. The older they get, the hairier, sweatier,

smellier, and messier they usually become. This presents a
problem for the sanitary woman. How many times have
you gotten dressed up for an evening of romance—armpits
waxed, eyebrows plucked, legs lotioned, lips glossed—only
to end up in bed with a man who hasn't changed his sheets
in six months and who leaves horrible, curly little pubes all
over his bathroom? You may be dating the sexiest man
alive at night, but even true love can't stop the morning
sun from shining on stained underwear.

What to do? This may be a question for an aesthetician,
not a doctor. However, there are medical reasons (and solu-
tions) for some sights and smells.

*In your practice, Harry, surely you see many hairy men. Why? Why
is it that women spend so much time shaving their pubic hair into
cute little designs, waxing it off, trimming it—while some men have
pubes that resemble Fangorn Forest. Is there any way to get guys to
trim down?*

☞ Actually, lots of guys are trimming their pubes these
days. Devices called "body trimmers" are selling like hot-
cakes—"body" in this case being a thinly disguised eu-
phemism for "pubic area." As many guys are learning,
"trimming the bushes around your deck makes your deck
look bigger." And if it appeals to women, so much the
better!

Meanwhile, a lot of guys think nothing of asking a
woman to shave or trim her pubic hair, but would be
surprised or indignant if the woman asked him to do
the same. That's a double standard that shouldn't be
tolerated. And maybe if more guys actually tried to
shave or trim their own genitals, they wouldn't so

blithely ask women to do it. These are very sensitive areas—and shaving them is a delicate business. Also, as any woman who has tried shaving will attest, the "nubs" stage of hair regrowth can be uncomfortable at best, painful at worst.

This all applies to guys, as well. Of all the parts of the male human body, the testicles are probably the most difficult to trim or shave. The skin of the testicles is in a difficult place to see clearly, it is wrinkled—meaning it's easy to injure if trying to shave—and it's both thin and extremely sensitive, making that "nubs" stage of hair regrowth even more uncomfortable for a guy than a woman.

Not that it's impossible to trim the hair on testicles—guys who get vasectomies are asked to shave their testicles prior to the procedure and few have any great difficulty doing so (though for most it's a novel experience). I tell such guys to consider doing the shaving after a hot bath, when the testicles are relaxed and the skin is more easily manipulated. Trimming the hair with a body trimmer or beard trimmer is another option and doesn't entail the same kind of uncomfortable regrowth period, because enough hair is left to prevent the "prickles." But still, it's tricky business, and a guy's gonna hurt himself if he's not careful. So if you do request a shave or trim from your partner, tell him to shower first and use a trimmer—or just be very careful.

How about unpleasant scents down there? A common one seems to be cabbage, and then there's the always-horrid cheese aroma.

☞ Guys who smell this way probably aren't circumcised. Strong cheesy or cabbagey odors from a penis are usually

related to a buildup of smegma, the whitish, waxlike substance that occurs naturally under the foreskin of an uncircumcised man. Regular cleaning of the penis by
retracting the foreskin and washing with soap and water
normally removes any buildup and keeps the penis
smelling normal.

If a guy's penis does smell bad, you should say something about it, and not just for your own sake. A buildup
of smegma can lead to an inflammation, called balanitis,
of the skin covering the head (glans) of the penis. Sometimes a man's foreskin is so tight it can't retract, a condition called phimosis. In such cases, the guy shouldn't try
to force the foreskin to retract because (a) it will hurt a
lot, and (b) it could damage the foreskin or glans. Phimosis and other types of foreskin malfunction can usually be corrected relatively easily if a guy gets prompt
medical attention.

*Got it. Easy to remember, too—cheesy cabbage isn't in danger of
becoming a cologne anytime soon. Are there any other bizarre
sights or smells that should trigger alarm?*

☞ Sure there are! As I just noted, healthy, clean male and
female genitals should not stink. They may have a dis-
tinctly musky odor, but it should be relatively light,
without strong sour, putrid, or cheesy odors. "Off" smells
most often mean a guy just needs to wash himself more
often, but they can also be signs of an infection or other
medical problem.

In terms of strange "sights," any type of open or
scabbed sore is an immediate warning sign, as are warts
and wartlike bumps. The colors of penises vary widely—

and not just because of racial differences. The penises of some white men are darker than you might expect. Also, curves and bends in an erect penis are not necessarily a bad sign, but keep an eye out for those that curve at an extreme angle. (See the discussion of Peyronie's disease on page 21.) As I've also discussed, it's normal for one of a man's testicles to hang lower than the other and for scrotal skin to be somewhat darker than the surrounding skin.

So you should definitely mention strange odors or a strange appearance. It might be awkward, but make sure he knows that you're doing it out of concern for him, not because you're just disgusted (and if you are just disgusted, pretend it's concern).

Also tell your partner if something feels strange. The testicles themselves should feel like very smooth, firm walnuts that slip around easily inside the scrotum. If you feel any kind of unusual lumps or hardness, speak up, since it could be testicular cancer, something many guys don't check for on a regular basis. Likewise, if you feel something like coiled string or ropes in the scrotum near one or both testicles, your guy probably has a condition called varicocele. This isn't a medical emergency, but it can hurt his fertility. Since varicoceles won't go away on their own and repair is not a complicated procedure, he should see a doctor fairly soon.

How about unsanitary sex practices?

☞ There's no danger at all from giving a guy fellatio after he's been in your vagina—even if you had an STI of some kind, you can't spread it to yourself.

But it's a very bad idea to get your mouth or vagina anywhere near a penis that has been in your rectum. The anus and rectum are simply swarming with bacteria, which can cause problems ranging from the unpleasant to the deadly if they are introduced to your vagina or mouth. There's nothing wrong with anal sex done with plenty of lubrication, gentleness (at least at first), and mutual consent. But it should be the last act of the play, so to speak.

How can women be sure that their partner's penis is clean, especially if he's gone to the bathroom recently? Guys' penises hang into the toilet, don't they? Gross.

☞ It's highly unlikely that his penis actually touches the toilet water. Not only would he have to bend in a weird and uncomfortable way, but it would probably gross out even the more troglodyte members of the gender. So relax and rely on your nose. A nice-smelling penis is a clean penis.

Can men get yeast infections?

☞ Yes, guys can get a yeast infection from sexual contact with a woman who has a vaginal yeast infection. The same yeast that causes vaginal infections in women can cause infections of the penis in men. It doesn't happen every time there's sexual contact, but if you have a UTI it's a good idea to abstain or get your guy to condom up. Signs and symptoms of a male yeast infection include a red rash, itching, and burning at the tip of the penis. Fortunately, most male yeast infections are easily treated with over-the-counter antifungal treatments, such as Monistat.

Why do some men have little bumpy, zitlike growths on their penis?

☞ Sometimes a hair will become ingrown and form a pim-
plelike bump. The same thing happens (with more regu-
larity) on men's faces, because when hairs are shaved
they are more easily tilted in the follicle, which makes
them grow sideways rather than up. This can be a real
hassle, especially for African Americans, whose hairs
tend to curl easily and thus get "misdirected" more often.

APPENDIX

The Male Package 101

LOOK AT A NAKED guy's privates and you see his penis and his scrotum. The penis will be circumcised (in which case the head, or glans, of the penis will be visible) or uncircumcised (in which case the glans is covered by the foreskin). Inside the scrotum are the two testes, also called the testicles. Each testicle is surrounded by layers of tissue, blood vessels, and muscles. The muscles allow the scrotum to contract or relax in response to cold or as part of the normal sexual response. Each testicle is a complicated structure that serves two functions: To make sperm and to make male sex hormones, particularly testosterone. Millions of sperm cells are produced daily in a healthy adult male. These cells mature as they move through a mass of tightly coiled tubes at the back of each testicle called the epididymis. When they leave the epididymis, sperm cells migrate up two thin tubes called the

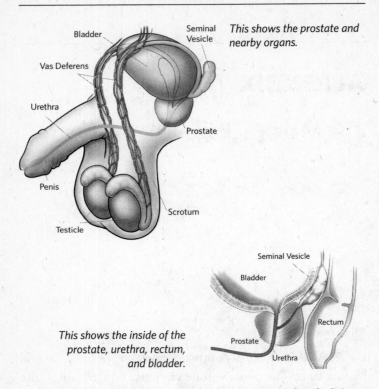

This shows the prostate and nearby organs.

Bladder
Seminal Vesicle
Vas Deferens
Urethra
Prostate
Penis
Scrotum
Testicle

Seminal Vesicle
Bladder
Rectum
Prostate
Urethra

This shows the inside of the prostate, urethra, rectum, and bladder.

vas deferens, which connect to the prostate gland. (Note: not "prostrate," which means lying horizontally.)

The prostate is about the size of a walnut and sits at the base of the bladder. Urine, stored in the bladder, passes through the middle of the prostate via a tube called the urethra. The urethra continues through the penis and carries urine during urination and semen during ejaculation (never both at the same time).

During orgasm, sperm in the vas deferens are propelled into the prostate gland, where they mix with a liquid containing sugar and enzymes. The seminal vesicles on the back of the bladder also provide liquid, and the resulting mixture is the milky white, slightly sweet substance called semen.

GLOSSARY

CIRCUMCISION—the surgical removal of the foreskin of the penis.

CRYPTORCHIDISM—a developmental defect marked by the failure of the testes to descend into the scrotum.

"DRY" OR RETROGRADE EJACULATION—when semen is forced backward into the bladder rather than out of the penis during orgasm. This occurs only when there is injury or a defect in the junction of the vas deferens and the urethra inside the prostate.

DYSPAREUNIA—the experience of pain during intercourse by either a man or a woman.

ELECTROEJACULATION—a procedure whereby a mild electric current is applied via a rectal probe to the prostate area, resulting in contraction of the pelvic muscles and ejaculation. Used to obtain semen from men who because of injury cannot ejaculate normally.

EPIDIDYMIS—a long, narrow, convoluted tube, part of the spermatic duct system, that lies on the rear portion of each testicle, connecting it to the vas deferens.

EPIDIDYMITIS—an infection of the epididymis.

FELLATIO—oral stimulation of the penis.

HPV (HUMAN PAPILLOMAVIRUS)—a virus with many subtypes, some of which can be transmitted during sex and can cause cell changes that increase the risk of certain cancers.

HYDROCELE—a noncancerous swelling of the scrotum caused by an abnormal accumulation of fluid due to injury or physiological defects.

HYPOSPADIAS—a congenital anomaly in which the urethral opening occurs not at the tip of the penis but some distance back from the tip on the underside of the penis.

IMPOTENCE—the inability to get or maintain an erection sufficient for intercourse (compare with *sterility*).

MICROPHALLUS—an abnormally small penis, typically less than 3 inches long when erect.

NOCTURNAL EMISSIONS—involuntary ejaculation while sleeping that may be accompanied by erotic dreams (also called "wet dreams").

NOCTURNAL PENILE TUMESCENCE TEST—a test that measures the expansion and contraction of the penis over the course of a night's sleep. If the test shows normal penile erections, the cause of impotence is likely to be psychological.

PARAPHILIA—a condition in which a person's sexual arousal and gratification depend on a fantasy theme of an unusual situation or object that becomes the principal focus of sexual behavior.

PERINEUM—the part of the body between the anus and the genitals.

PEYRONIE'S DISEASE—an abnormal curvature of an erect penis that may interfere with intercourse.

PHIMOSIS—an abnormal constriction of the foreskin that prevents it from being drawn back to uncover the head of the penis.

PREMATURE EJACULATION—ejaculation that regularly occurs sooner than desired, either before or shortly after penetration, in many cases causing distress to one or both partners.

PRIAPISM—an abnormally prolonged erection, which poses a significant risk for permanent damage to the penis.

PROSTATE—the walnut-sized gland at the base of the bladder that contributes part of the seminal fluid and that participates in propelling semen from the penis during ejaculation.

PROSTATECTOMY—surgical removal of the prostate or a portion thereof.

PROSTATITIS—infection of the prostate.

SMEGMA—the cheesy substance normally secreted under the foreskin; it is typically washed off during normal bathing.

STERILITY—the inability to conceive a child (compare with *impotence*).

VARICOCELES—abnormally enlarged veins in the scrotum, which can impair fertility if not treated.

VASECTOMY—surgical cutting of the vas deferens to make a man sterile.

FINDING HELP

Dr. Harry Fisch
Professor of clinical urology, Columbia University; director, The Male Reproductive Center at Columbia University Medical Center/New York Presbyterian Hospital; adjunct professor of urology, Medical University of South Carolina; author, *The Male Biological Clock*
944 Park Avenue, New York, NY 10028
212-879-0800
www.harryfisch.com

Dr. Marianne J. Legato
Professor of clinical medicine, Columbia University Medical Center/New York Presbyterian Hospital; director and founder of the Partnership for Gender-Specific Medicine; author of *Why Men Never Remember and Women Never Forget, Eve's Rib: The Groundbreaking Guide to Women's Health, What Women Need to Know,* and *The Female Heart: The Truth About Women and Heart Disease*
962 Park Avenue, New York, NY 10028
212-737-6306

Dr. Benjamin Lewis
Associate professor of medicine/cardiology, Columbia University
Medical Center/New York Presbyterian Hospital
16 East 60th Street, New York, NY 10022
212-326-8425

Dr. Jon LaPook
Associate professor of medicine/gastroenterology, Columbia
University Medical Center/New York Presbyterian Hospital
16 East 60th Street, New York, NY 10022
212-326-8405

American Association of Sex Educators, Counselors, and Therapists
PO Box 5488, Richmond, VA 23220-0488
www.aasect.org

American Diabetes Association
1701 North Beauregard Street, Alexandria, VA 22311
1-800-DIABETES
www.diabetes.org

Sexual Function Health Council, American Foundation for Urologic Disease
1128 North Charles Street, Baltimore, MD 21201
800-433-4215 or 410-468-1800
impotence@afud.org
www.impotence.org

American Infertility Association
666 Fifth Avenue, Suite 278, New York, NY 10103
888-917-3777
info@americaninfertility.org

American Society for Reproductive Medicine
1209 Montgomery Highway, Birmingham, AL 35216-2809
205-978-5000
www.asrm.org (Note: includes a "find a doctor" service for locating fertility specialists in a given area)

American Urological Association
1120 North Charles Street, Baltimore, MD 21201
410-727-1100
aua@auanet.org / www.auanet.org

RESOLVE: The National Infertility Association
1310 Broadway, Somerville, MA 02144
888-623-0744
info@resolve.org, www.resolve.org

Dr. Natan Bar-Chama
Director, The Center for Male Reproductive Health
The Mount Sinai School of Medicine
Department of Urology
5 East 98th Street, Box 1272
New York, NY 10029
212-241-7443
natan.bar-chama@mountsinai.org

Dr. Ridwan Shabsigh
Director, Division of Urology, Maimonides Medical Center; professor of clinical urology, Columbia University; author of *Sensational Sex in 7 Easy Steps: The Proven Plan for Enhancing Your Sexual Function and Achieving Optimum Health*
718-283-7746
www.shabsigh7steps.com.

Dr. Peter Schlegel
Chairman and professor of urology, Cornell University/New
York Presbyterian Hospital
Starr 900, Department of Urology
New York Presbyterian/Weill Cornell
525 East 68th Street, New York, NY 10021
212-746-5491
www.cornellurology.com/infertility/physicians.shtml

Dr. Marc Goldstein
Director, The Center for Male Reproductive Medicine; professor
of urology, Cornell University/New York Presbyterian Hospital
Starr 900, Department of Urology
New York Presbyterian/Weill Cornell
525 East 68th Street, New York, NY 10021
212-746-5470
www.cornellurology.com/infertility/physicians.shtml

Dr. Michael A. Perelman
Codirector, Human Sexuality Program, Cornell University/New
York Presbyterian Hospital
70 East 77th Street, Suite 1C, New York, NY 10021
212-570-5000
Perelman@earthlink.net

NOTES

1. Awwad Z, Abu-Hijleh M, Basri S, Shegam N, Murshidi M, Ajlouni K. Penile measurements in normal adult Jordanians and in patients with erectile dysfunction. *Int J Impot Res.* 2005 Mar–Apr;17(2):191–5.

2. Wessells H, Lue TF, McAninch JW. Penile length in the flaccid and erect states: guidelines for penile augmentation. *Journal of Urology.* 1996 Sep;156(3):995–7.

3. Masters WH, Johnson VE. *Human Sexual Response.* 1966. Little, Brown & Co. Boston. Page 192.

4. This is an extrapolation from the urological recommendations that only men with a stretched penile length shorter than 7.5 centimeters should seek penile enhancement surgery. The erect penis is, of course, slightly longer (but not by much) than a stretched penis. See: Wessells H, Lue TF, McAninch JW. Penile length in the flaccid and erect states: guidelines for penile augmentation. *J Urol.* 1996 Sep;156(3):995–7.

5. Orakwe JC, Ogbuagu BO, Ebuh GU. Can physique and gluteal size predict penile length in adult Nigerian men? *West Afr J Med.* 2006 Jul–Sep;25(3):223–5.

6. Masters WH, Johnson VE. *Human Sexual Response*. 1966. Little, Brown & Co. Boston. Page 192.

7. Griffin G. *Penis Size and Enlargement: Facts, Fallacies, and Proven Methods*. Aptos, CA: Hourglass, 1995.

8. Shamloul R. Treatment of men complaining of short penis. *Urology* 2005;65(6):1183–5.

9. Kinsey AC, Pomeroy WB, Martin CE. *Sexual Behavior in the Human Male*. Philadelphia: W.B. Saunders Co., 1948.

10. Masters WH, Johnson VE. *Human Sexual Response*. 1966. Little, Brown & Co. Boston. Page 193.

11. Hamilton, T. *Skin Flutes and Velvet Gloves*. New York: St. Martin's Press, 2002.

12. Orakwe JC, Ogbuagu BO, Ebuh GU. Can physique and gluteal size predict penile length in adult Nigerian men? *West Afr J Med.* 2006 Jul–Sep;25(3):223–5.

13. This and the other information about Peyronie's disease is adapted from information on the website of the National Institute for Diabetes and Digestive and Kidney Disorders, NIH. Available at: http://kidney.niddk.nih.gov/kudiseases/pubs/peyronie/index.htm. Accessed 5/12/07.

14. Masters WH, Johnson VE. *Human Sexual Response*. 1966. Little, Brown & Co. Boston. Pages 198–199.

15. Stulhofer A. How (Un)Important Is Penis Size for Women with Heterosexual Experience? *Archives of Sexual Behavior* 2006;35(1):5.

16. Dabbs JM, LaRue D, Williams PM. Testosterone and occupational choice: Actors, ministers, and other men. *Journal of Personality and Social Psychology* 1990;59:1261–1265.

17. Rhoden EL, Morgentaler A. Risks of testosterone-replacement therapy and recommendations for monitoring. *New England Journal of Medicine* 2004;350:482–492.

18. Demark-Wahnefried W, et al. Serum androgens: associations with prostate cancer risk and hair patterning. *Journal of Andrology*. 1998 Sep–Oct;19(5):631.

19. Bhasin S, Buckwalter JG. Testosterone supplementation in older men: a rational idea whose time has not yet come. *J Androl.* 2001;22:718–731.

20. Brambilla DJ, O'Donnel AB, Matsumoto AM, McKinlay JM. Lack of seasonal variation in serum sex hormone levels in middle-aged to older men in the Boston area. *Journal of Clinical Endocrinology & Metabolism.* Vol. 92, No. 11, 4224–4229.

21. Fisch H. *The Male Biological Clock.* New York: Free Press, 2005.

22. Jones JC, Barlow DH. Self-reported frequency of sexual urges, fantasies, and masturbatory fantasies in heterosexual males and females. *Arch Sex Behav.* 1990 Jun;19(3):269–79.

23. Feldman HA, Goldstein I, Hatzichristou DG, Krane RJ, McKinlay JB. Impotence and its medical and psychosocial correlates: results of the Massachusetts Male Aging Study. *J Urol.* 1994;151:54–61.

24. Atwood JD, Schwartz L. Cybersex: The new affair; treatment considerations. *Journal of Couple and Relationship Therapy* 2002;1(3):37–56.

25. Diagnostic and Statistical Manual of Mental Disorders, Fourth Edition, Text Revision. Washington, D.C.: American Psychiatric Association, 2000.

26. Seidel HM, Ball JW, Dains JE, Benedict GW. *Mosby's Guide to Physical Examination,* 4th Ed. St. Louis: Mosby, Inc., 1999.

27. Masters WH, Johnson VE. *Human Sexual Response.* 1966. Little, Brown & Co. Boston. Page 207.

28. Mayo Clinic Health Information website. Available at: www.mayoclinic.com/health/hydrocele/DS00617/DSECTION =7. Accessed 9/17/07.

29. Masters WH, Johnson VE. *Human Sexual Response.* 1966. Little, Brown & Co. Boston. Page 198.

30. Laumann E, Gagnon JH, Michael RT, and Michaels S. *The Social Organization of Sexuality: Sexual Practices in the United States.* Chicago: University of Chicago Press, 1994.

31. www.jackinworld.com/expert/index.html.

32. Kinsey AC, *Sexual Behavior in the Human Male.* Bloomington, IN: Indiana University Press, 1953.

33. Hamilton T. *Skin Flutes and Velvet Gloves*. 2002. St. Martin's Press. New York. Page 55.

34. Schover LR, Thomas AJ. *Overcoming Male Infertility: Understanding Its Causes and Treatments*. 2000. John Wiley & Sons Inc. New York. Page 36.

35. Masters WH, Johnson VE. *Human Sexual Response*. 1966. Little, Brown & Co. Boston. Page 216.

36. Jiang M, Xin J, Zou Q, Shen JW. A research on the relationship between ejaculation and serum testosterone level in men. *J Zhejiang Univ. Sci.* 2003;4(2):236–240.

37. Cohen A, Wong ML, Resnick D. Localized seminal plasma protein hypersensitivity. *Allergy Asthma Proc.* 2004 Jul–Aug;25(4):261–2.

38. Handelsman DJ, Conway AJ, Radonic I, Turtle JR. Prevalence, testicular function and seminal parameters in men with sperm antibodies. *Clin Reprod Fertil.* 1983;2(1):39–45.

39. Fisch H, Braun S. *The Male Biological Clock*. 2005. The Free Press. New York. Page 3.

40. Patrick DL, et al. Premature ejaculation: An observational study of men and their partners. *J Sex Med.* 2005;2:358–367.

41. Kinsey, AC, et al. 1948/1998. *Sexual Behavior in the Human Male*. Philadelphia: W.B. Saunders; Bloomington, IN: Indiana U. Press. Page 580.

42. Diamond J. Everything *Else* You Ever Wanted to Know About Sex. *Discover*, April 1985, p. 73, column 1.

43. Chang J. *The Tao of Love and Sex*. E.P. Dutton, New York. 1977. Page 21.

44. Smith TW. *American Sexual Behavior: Trends, Socio-Demographic Differences, and Risk Behavior*. National Opinion Research Center, University of Chicago. GSS Topical Report No. 25. Updated March 2006.

45. Marieb EN. *Human Anatomy and Physiology*, 2nd Ed. 1992. Benjamin Cummings Publishing Co., Redwood City, CA. Page 501.

46. Kinsey AC, et al. 1953/1998. *Sexual Behavior in the Human Female*. Philadelphia: W.B. Saunders; Bloomington, IN: Indiana U. Press. Page 664.

47. Cooper A, Scherer C, Boies S, Gordon B. Sexuality on the Internet: From sexual exploration to pathological expression. 1999. Vol. 30(2), pp. 154–164.

48. Masters WH, Johnson VE. *Human Sexual Response*. 1966. Little, Brown & Co. Boston. Page 285.

49. Marieb EN. *Human Anatomy and Physiology*, 2nd Ed. 1992. Benjamin Cummings Publishing Co., Redwood City, CA. Page 967.

50. University of California at Santa Barbara SexInfo website. www.soc.ucsb.edu/sexinfo/?article=hKjl. Accessed 8/21/07.

51. Chang J. *The Tao of Love and Sex*. New York: E.P. Dutton, 1977.

52. Halvorsen BL, Holte K, Myhrstad MC, et al. A Systematic Screening of Total Antioxidants in Dietary Plants. *Journal of Nutrition* 2002;132:461–471.

53. Young S. The Subtle Side of Sex. *New Scientist* 1993, August 14, 24–27.

54. Berger GS, Goldstein M, Fuerst M. *The Couple's Guide to Fertility*, 3rd Ed. New York: Broadway Books, 2001.

55. Eskenazi B, Wyrobek AJ, Sloter E, Kidd SA, Moore L, Young S. The association of age and semen quality in healthy men. *Human Reproduction* 2003;18(2):447–454.

56. Karabinus DS. Chromatin structural changes in sperm after scrotal insulation of Holstein bulls. *J Androl.*, Vol. 18, No. 5. September/October 1997.

57. Levin RJ. The physiology of sexual arousal in the human female: a recreational and procreational synthesis. *Arch Sex Behav.* 2002 Oct;31(5):405–11.

58. Ménézo YJ, Hazout A, Panteix G, et al. Antioxidants to reduce sperm DNA fragmentation: an unexpected adverse effect. *Reprod Biomed Online* 2007;14(4):418–421.

59. Thayer RE. *The Origin of Everyday Moods*. New York: Oxford University Press, 1996.

60. Shabsigh R, Rowland D. The *Diagnostic and Statistical Manual of Mental Disorders*, Fourth Edition, Text Revision as an Appropriate Diagnostic for Premature Ejaculation. *J Sex Med.* 2007;4:1468–1478.

61. Wilson GT, Lawson DM. Expectancies, alcohol, and sexual arousal in male social drinkers. *J Abnormal Psych.* 1976;85: 587–594.

62. *Marijuana and Medicine: Assessing the Science Base.* Institute of Medicine, National Academy of Sciences, 1999.

63. Jackson AL, Murphy LL. Role of the hypothalamic-pituitary-adrenal axis in the suppression of luteinizing hormone release by delta-9-tetrahydrocannabinol. *Neuroendocrinology* 1997. 65:446–452.

64. Vale J. Benign prostatic hyperplasia and erectile dysfunction—is there a link? *Curr Med Res Opin.* 2000;16 Suppl. 1:s63–7.

65. Feldman HA, Goldstein I, Hatzichristou DG, Krane RJ, McKinlay JB. Impotence and its medical and psychosocial correlates: results of the Massachusetts Male Aging Study. *J Urol.* 1994;151:54–61.

66. Berman JR, Berman LA, Toler SM, Gill J, Haughie S; Sildenafil Study Group. Safety and efficacy of sildenafil citrate for the treatment of female sexual arousal disorder: a double-blind, placebo controlled study. *J Urol.* 2003 Dec;170(6 Pt. 1):2333–8.

67. Edwards S, Carne C. Oral sex and transmission of non-viral STIs. *Sexually Transmitted Infections* 1998;74(2):95–100.

68. Koutsky L. Epidemiology of genital human papillomavirus infection. *American Journal of Medicine* 1997;102(5A):3–8.

69. Weinstock H, Berman S, Cates Jr. W. Sexually transmitted diseases among American youth: incidence and prevalence estimates, 2000. *Perspectives on Sexual and Reproductive Health* 2004;36(1):6–10.

ACKNOWLEDGMENTS

FIRST things first. I'd like to thank my girl friends, especially my oldest ones: Katie Leeman, Jessica Ross, and Elizabeth Brusie, whom I've known since my sole experience with dating was kissing my New Kids on the Block pillowcase. Together we've navigated the often alarming waters of male/female relations and have only gotten better and more smolderingly good-looking with age. Flipping through our junior high school yearbook, it's amazing we managed to date at all. Ain't life grand?

To Lisa Johnson, Liz LaRocca, Sara Share, Stevie Groopman, Jesse Achtenberg, Sharon King, Jess Bricker, Adam Perlmutter, Sarah DeWitt, Meghann Marshall, Claudia Lee, Jenny and John Kissko, Rianka Mohan, Vicky Lucas, Daniela

Constantino, Brad Szathmary, Jenn Lee, Alison Raymond, and Auntie Ei—terrific friends, all of them, and completely okay with my lack of boundaries in the interest of research . . . or in the course of daily life. Extra-special love to my sisters-in-law, Joy Lapseritis and Diane Hart, for being great family and also good friends. And I owe an immense debt of gratitude to Dr. Stephen Stein, who has an enormous influence on my life.

To Gail Ross, for luring me into this project, for being a kick-ass lady, and for being so amazingly supportive of all my professional endeavors. To Howard Yoon, for his candor, sense of humor, and for just being so intelligent all the time. To office goddess Jennifer Manguera, for mailing those checks UPS Next-Day. To Steve Braun, who did an enormous amount of medical research and writing behind the scenes, and of course to Harry Fisch, for bringing this idea to fruition. To Lindsey Moore, our editor, for championing Harry's idea in the first place.

Finally, I'd like to thank my grandparents, parents, and my brother, Matthew. Not much is worth doing in life without a supportive family. My brother is my best friend and one of my favorite writers. (Although if he grows up to write a book about vaginas, I might cry.) As for my parents, they have a terrific sense of humor and took this latest career turn in stride. All the late nights I've spent working on this book have proved more than worth it, if only to hear my mother say: "Are you done with that penis book yet?!" And last but definitely not least: I'd like to thank my husband, Brian Lapseritis, whose manhood is sufficiently intact not to be offended or frightened that I'm coauthoring a book on men's penises.

Some men would file for divorce or join the Witness Protection Program, but not Brian. It takes a special guy to be supportive of such an endeavor. He's also asking that I emphasize that none of the questions contained in this book have anything to do with him whatsoever. Especially the part about bad personal hygiene. I'm a lucky girl.

—KARA BASKIN

WRITING this book was very difficult for many different reasons. On numerous occasions, I consulted my friends and colleagues for advice and guidance. I want to thank Dr. Natan Bar-Chama, director of the Male Reproductive Center at the Mount Sinai Hospital in New York; Dr. Ridwan Shabsigh, who is the chairman of the Department of Urology at Maimonides Medical Center; Dr. Michael Perelman, the codirector of the Human Sexuality Program of the New York Presbyterian Hospital; Dr. Benjamin Lewis and Dr. Jon LaPook, two extraordinary physicians in the Department of Medicine, Columbia University Medical Center; Dr. Marianne Legato, who founded the Partnership for Gender-Specific Medicine at Columbia University College of Physicians and Surgeons; and Dr. Grace Hyun, Dr. Kimberly Cooper, Dr. Debra Fromer, Dr. Erica Lambert, Dr. Sarah Lambert, and the residents of the Department of Urology at Columbia University.

I want to thank my assistant of the last 15 years, Madelon Makowski, and the nurses and staff of the operating and recovery rooms at the Allen Pavilion of Columbia University Medical Center/New York Presbyterian Hospital.

The actual writing of this book would never have been possible without Stephen Braun, who is phenomenal. Thank you to Kara Baskin for providing the female voice for this book. And to Howard Yoon and Gail Ross, my literary agents, for thinking that this book could make a difference.

I especially want to thank my family: my children, David, Melissa, and Sam; and my wife, Karen, to whom I owe it all.

HARRY FISCH, M.D.

INDEX

ABOUT THE AUTHORS

DR. HARRY FISCH is one of the nation's foremost urologists. He is a professor of urology at Columbia University (where he was recently named Teacher of the Year), and the director of the Male Reproductive Center at Columbia University Medical Center/New York Presbyterian Hospital. Dr. Fisch lectures constantly and has published numerous articles on male infertility and men's health, most recently in the prestigious *Journal of the American Medical Association*. His 2004 book, *The Male Biological Clock*, was called "fascinating and well-written" by Bob Bazell of NBC News and "blunt and informative" by Amazon.com. He is widely recognized as an expert in his field, having been quoted in publications such as the *New York Times* and *The Economist* and appearing on the *Today* show, the CBS *Evening News*, *Good Morning America*, *60 Minutes*, *20/20*, CNN, and others. Dr. Fisch has treated countless men in his private practice.

KARA BASKIN is the editor of *Lola*, the *Boston Globe*'s lifestyle magazine for women. A former editor for *The New Republic*, she has written for *Slate*, the *New York Observer*, the *Washington Post*, *The Washingtonian*, the *Boston Phoenix*, and NPR.org, and coauthored Avalon's Moon Metro travel series on Washington, D.C. She has collaborated on many nonfiction books and is a frequent public speaker on women's health issues.